A Month Among the Vines

Since becoming an Anglican priest in 1978, Rev Andrew Procter has been incumbent in a Yorkshire Dales village, an inner-city suburb and a village just within the M25. He has always been dedicated to getting in among people: as a young curate he once spent two weeks working on a car production line in order to find out more about the life of his parishioners; in 2000 he donned a monastic robe and spent a month walking the Yorkshire Dales, carrying no money, sharing the Gospel with people he met. He is a poet, an accredited counsellor, a keen gardener and cricket enthusiast.

In 2003 Andrew and his wife Elizabeth, a psychiatrist, co-authored "Exploring God", a study course designed to help people discover the God within them. They have four grown-up children and live in Kent.

*To Liz
with gratitude for your faithful
listening
with love   Faye*

£1.50

A Month Among the Vines

*Daily devotions based on time shared with a
L'Arche community in France*

Andrew Procter

*Blessings,
Andrew*

A Redemptorist Publication

Published by Redemptorist Publications

ISBN 0 85231 309 8

A catalogue record for this book is available from the British Library.

Cover Design: Arcus Design
Layout: Rosemarie Pink

Printed by Cambridge University Press Ltd.

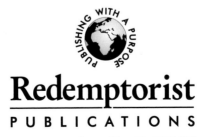

Redemptorist
PUBLICATIONS

Alphonsus House Chawton Hampshire GU34 3HQ
Telephone 01420 88222 Fax 01420 88805
www.rpbooks.co.uk email rp@rpbooks.co.uk

I dedicate this book to Hervé Sheptou – about the finest man I know

Contents

Acknowledgements

Many people have helped me bring this book into being. I would like to thank them here.

In chronological order they are my fellow members of our church writers' group, without whom I would have given up writing long before starting this book. I would like especially to name the longest serving members: Hilda Brown, Penny Culliford, Lorna Kahan and Tim Jacob. I would also like to thank Chris Waddington, Jeannette Phillips, Paul Moseley, Kath Davis, Maggie Graham and Dorothy White who kindly piloted the first draft. Their comments were invaluable and without exception followed in producing the second draft. My daughter, Kate Mendez, whose comments on the second draft were as necessarily ruthless as only one's grown-up daughter's can be; my daughter, Emily Wingfield and Sr Gertrude RGS who began then to pray this book into the public domain and are still at it; the staff at Redemptorist Publications, notably Marguerite Hutchinson, Trish Wilson, Caroline Hodgson and Andrew Lyon; the staff at L'Arche UK Head Office, especially John Peet, Judith Ellis and David Winpenny; the leaders of L'Arche France, particularly Erik Pillet, Louis Pilote and Antoine de Terves; The Rt Revd Richard Chartres, the Bishop of London, for his kind foreword, and those who gave the book their celebrity endorsements.

I want, at this point, to thank the leaders of L'Arche UK for their co-operation in the preparation of this book. It was a great relief to me that they liked it and were prepared to support it. They have asked me to say, though, that the rural situation and life of the community at La Rebellerie which I describe is not typical of most L'Arche communities in the UK, which are mostly urban with an emphasis on integration with local community care provision.

Of course I need to say that, whatever becomes of this book, I will ever remain indebted to all who make life at La Rebellerie what it is and for letting me share it with them for a little while. Even more incalculable is what I owe to my wife Elizabeth. She has not failed me as I worked on this book or in anything else.

Andrew Procter

Foreword

Jean Vanier is among the very few authentic prophets of our own day. In founding L'Arche communities around the world, he has provided direct entry into the mystery that we find the more we go beyond ourselves in service of one another.

In L'Arche communities, people with various kinds of learning disabilities live full lives as members of the community, which is always engaged with the world around it.

As someone who had the privilege of living with a brother with severe disabilities I have admired the work of L'Arche for many years. I know first hand the gifts that are to be found in such communities. In past years I have often directed brainy, emotionally starved ordinands to spend time as an assistant in a L'Arche community. My experience is that they rarely emerge without a much clearer insight into their vocation and with an increase of joy.

Andrew Procter has witnessed the L'Arche phenomenon in France. His report *A Month Among the Vines* is both moving and humorous and breathes the spirit of L'Arche itself. He distils some very simple but deep wisdom from his sojourn in L'Arche and I believe that if this account is approached with an open mind and a prayerful heart, the reader will also come closer to an understanding experience of the healing power of the love of God.

The Rt Revd & Rt Hon Richard Chartres
Bishop of London

INTRODUCTION

E very few years, if you are a member of the clergy, they give you time off work for good behaviour. It's called a "sabbatical" and you can go off and do something different from parish life in the hope it will enrich your ministry.

When my sabbatical was due I knew I wanted to spend at least part of it experiencing the life of a L'Arche community if I could. L'Arche (which is French for "the ark") was founded in 1964 when two men, Jean Vanier and Father Thomas Philippe, invited two other men, Raphael Simi and Philippe Seux, who had learning disabilities, to share life in community together. They had no thoughts of it at the time, but from this small beginning has now grown a worldwide movement. Jean Vanier is known internationally as a Christian writer and thinker of great humility and power. It was in reading his books that I first came by the inspiring message of L'Arche. It struck a chord with me. Vanier spoke of the aridity of constantly seeking success:

> In richer countries life is dominated
> by constant competition,
> by the struggle for success and power.
> In Canada I saw a sign in a classroom:
> "It is a crime not to excel."
> Each one of us must succeed;

if we do not, we will have no status in society,
no work, no home.
We must win the prize or else be discarded.
So we learn to harden our hearts and fight and struggle
to be first ...
But many people who appear powerful and successful
can also feel worthless deep inside themselves.
They have money, power, education, status,
but they lack what is essential:
a heart that is free and loving ...
They too feel they belong to no one.
They feel that terrible pain of being unable to love,
of isolation,
unable to break out of their shell ...
(from *The Broken Body*, by Jean Vanier)

I felt I related deeply with that, even as a priest. I had striven for success over so long. I was jaded and embittered and emotionally isolated. I wanted to taste the "qualities of welcome, wonderment, spontaneity and directness" which the L'Arche charter attributes to those with learning disabilities. I had twice managed to spend short times with L'Arche communities whilst still engaged in parish ministry and found the experience quite profound if all too brief. And so, when the opportunity came, I was off to the West of France for time at La Rebellerie, a working vineyard and well-established L'Arche community. It was a crazy time of hard work, hard learning, many mistakes. As the charter also says, "weakness and vulnerability in a person, far from being an obstacle to union with God, can foster it. It is often through weakness recognised and accepted that the liberating love of God is revealed." That was certainly true for me. I found my time there one of much weakness yet of deep rediscovery of my God as a God of love. And it was all so comical and human and often such fun.

Near the end of my month in the community I was praying in my room (which when not in use for accommodation was the house's *orotoire* or prayer room) about how to hold on to the lessons I had been so privileged to learn. It seemed to come to me in a flash: "write it up as a devotional." So this is what I have done. I have divided up my experiences at L'Arche into a month's worth of daily reflections. Each one describes something about my life as part of the community. Then I have added a thought for the day which links the reflection to a facet of our Christian faith. I have also added a prayer for use either as it stands or as an entrée into further prayers of the readers' own. And I have chosen a Bible passage or two along the same theme. Finally, I have chosen a particular Bible verse or part of a verse for meditation.

Each daily section is designed for something like ten minutes' worth of devotional time. Reading my description of life at L'Arche should take about five minutes, the Bible passages another three minutes or so and that leaves time to read the prayer and take a couple of minutes for meditation and reflection. These are minimum times, of course, with busy people in mind. I would hope the reader with the leisure to use them for longer would be able to extend these suggested guidelines and feel further nourished still by the spirit of L'Arche.

DAY ONE
The Journey There

"God chose the foolish things of the world to shame the wise"

Imust admit, I was looking forward to my journey over to the community at La Rebellerie. I fancied getting off the domestic leash a bit and being something of an urbane, international traveller. I had a slim new briefcase and matching grip bag. I wore chinos and an open-necked shirt. I wanted to cut a bit of a dash, driving footloose and fancy free through the lanes of France, dining at a charming old hotel overnight, speaking effortless French to the patron (hotelier) and feeling cosmopolitan and debonair and dashing for once in my life.

But it was not to be. Arriving a little late at Newhaven I was handed a leaflet informing me of various things without which it was illegal to drive in France. There were draconian on-the-spot fines and impoundments for failure to possess these essentials. I had none of them. So I dutifully went into a little shed of a shop that was there for mugs like me and paid out for sixty-five quid's worth of stuff, fretting all the while that the queue in which I had left the car would be waved onto the ship in my absence, and I would cause an embarrassing hold up. I flopped back into my seat in a lather with my fire extinguisher, warning triangle and first-aid kit all over my lap just in time to be waved on board. Once over the ramp there was a tight, steep spiral to be driven more or less in the darkness, bumper to bumper with the other cars – more sweat. When I finally parked my hands were shaking.

I was no less jittery on the crossing. I suppose I was nervous about the month ahead. I kept getting up and changing my seat, starting different books and ending up reading the courtesy copies of the *Daily Mail* from cover to cover. I also ate too much, a regular failing when travelling, ending up by ordering a paella at the last minute. It proved to be a wretched, congealed microwave meal as tasteless as polystyrene, and I had to cram it down as we were being called to return to our vehicles.

At my hotel, more ignominy awaited. I addressed the patron in my best French, asking where I might park the car. His little droopy moustache drooped rather more on hearing me and his great tired eyes accepted just a little more pain in a painful life. He answered me in English.

"M'sieur may park in the garages opposite. Will M'sieur require dinner?"

It was now nearly ten at night, but I did so want a characterful French dinner, and didn't they eat late in France? So, with a gulp, I said yes and realised from his expression that I had just caused even more pain.

"Very well, M'sieur", he said in a tone that spoke volumes.

When I entered the restaurant, the final diners were leaving. It was a quiet, mid-week evening. The air hung with coffee and cigar smoke. As I sat down, not even that hungry, a young waiter, thin as a blade, dumped a basket of bread down in front of me with a look of pure vitriol. Plainly this rosbif had just caused the staff to have to work an extra hour. I ate my way through five courses with each one whisked away the moment it was finished and the following one brought out immediately. I did get to sit upstairs by my open shutters soothing myself with a cigar. At least the French had no qualms about smoking in bedrooms.

The next morning was cold and rainy; I got lost getting out of the small town. I got lost in the ring road system around Le Mans, making circuits of the city as if I thought it was the famous racing track. I got lost in Angers and had to make an inarticulate mobile phone call in French to the community explaining that I was to be late. I finally got there; sweaty and done in, two and a half hours late, dying for the loo. My first encounter with my hosts was to ask breathlessly for "la toilette" and disappear off down the corridor. As you must agree, every inch the urbane, international traveller.

Thought for the Day

When did you last look a proper silly? Days? Months? Years? If it's a long time ago, maybe check out if you are not living a bit on the safe, unadventurous side. Because doing stuff for God has a way of letting you look foolish. He takes you into new places where you stumble around and make mistakes. What you had fancied as an impressive mission dumps you on your backside. When you thought you would be so good, you just look daft – at least at the start. That's a hallmark of God's hand in things. There's a saying: "Give me a young man who has brains enough to make a fool of himself." I think maybe God says that to us all at times.

Prayer

Lord, I hate looking foolish, but, if I'm honest, I care too much for my precious dignity. You had no dignity at all left to you at the end. I know that. Please help me to be prepared to look foolish where it's part of your calling. And, (I know I am going to regret praying this) do something in my life to stir me up from living within my dignity the whole time. Amen.

Bible Passages
Exodus 4:10-16; 5:1-4. 19-23
Moses frightened of looking stupid, then looking stupid.

Joshua 7:2-9
Joshua learning from looking stupid.

2 Samuel 6:12-23
King David prepared to lose his dignity.

1 Corinthians 4:8-13
Paul happy to be a fool for Christ's sake.

For Meditation
"God chose the foolish things of the world to shame the wise."
(1 Corinthians 1:27)

DAY TWO

The Foyer

*"When my spirit grows faint within me,
it is you who know my way!"*

My arrival had been to the central community buildings at La Rebellerie. Georges, one of the senior members, took me over to the foyer (community house) in which I was to live. It had its own name, "La Croisée". It looked gorgeous from the outside. It had a low-slung, red-tiled roof. The tiles were each like half an old-fashioned plant pot and made long half-circle rows. Incredibly attractive. And it had cream walls. There was nobody about so Georges said just to kill time for a bit. I sat at a table under the trees in the garden and wrote letters home saying how idyllic it was going to be. I imagined meals out there in the sun. If it was cold there was the beamed main room with a fireplace in the corner and a large wooden dining table twisted with age. My room was the "oratoire" (prayer room), converted to a bedroom for my short stay. It, too, had a deep fireplace into which had been placed a large section of a tree trunk. On this was an array of attractive candles and a couple of icons. There were nice texts and devotional posters around the walls. My bed was a low-lying put-you-up bed in a corner. There was a low sofa affair as well. All the colours were subdued. I felt it was going to be a place of seclusion and peace. My heart lifted when I saw it.

In fact I was to have a difficult time in that foyer. It wasn't as clean as it looked. There was plenty of grime when you got close up. The showers only worked if you held the shower rose over your own head, and then not very well. The attractive-looking wooden settles in the lounge were abominable to sit on. And the flies! My own room, which I had envisaged as a haven, was a mecca for them. I got a shock after coming in from my first long hard day in the vine fields. I opened my door and immediately set a-buzzing some hundreds of flies. Repulsed, I picked up my sponge bag to make for the shower. A swarm of flies eddied out from it – apparently they seek damp places. My clothes were covered too. All through my stay I was to do battle with them. I pretty soon gave up leaving my large window open, though it made the room stiflingly hot, but they still seemed to get in by the score. I took to avoiding that otherwise lovely room. But I had to go to bed. My every move as I undressed was reflected by the buzzing of disturbed flies. Only when I finally laid down did they cease and settle in black dots all over my white walls. They seemed like grumpy bedmates in a dormitory, buzzing at me to lie still and go to sleep.

In fact I never could get comfortable somehow in that place. My one solace was to ring home from the office, which was clean and tidy and relatively fly free. Then the handset broke and I had to crouch on the tiled floor in the dark corridor outside the kitchen door to use the other phone, with people clomping past all the time and treading on me. After a fortnight of it I was ready to come home. I remember telling Elizabeth so one night and sensing her groan inwardly at yet another volte-face from her mercurial husband. (She was quite enjoying her month's sabbatical too – from me). But something happened to save me. The final night before I was due to leave for a quick visit home for my daughter's graduation ceremony was the 14th July, the day on which the storming of the Bastille is commemorated – a big night in the French year. I had been out and got back to find the place deserted but for someone I had not met before. Everybody else was out at a fireworks party. She was called Audrey. She was about thirty. And we had a good conversation. It was as simple as that. We sat on those settles and talked. About important things. For some reason I seemed able to raise my French above the level of banal commonplaces. It was so pleasant to be doing what I do best – listening to people talk out their troubles and supporting them. After a couple of hours we had a tisane, which I discovered to be ideal after such an evening. And, I realised with a shock, I had been comfortable! Not just in my body but in my spirit. I had somehow arrived. It felt warm and soothing. I knew then that I would return and complete my month.

The following morning was brightly sunny. I found myself sat on the bench outside the front door surrounded by a laughing group who now seemed friends. I smoked a cigar and drank in the ambience of belonging. I had a light heart. Something difficult had been overcome. Some process had been gone through, which had been worth the discomfort.

Thought for the Day

Think over your experience to date. Can you spot any "breakthroughs" similar to mine in the foyer? Has God taken you to the wire before you made it to the other side of something? Have there been times when a moment of despair about something has proven also to be the moment of release or victory? This could be in matters small like mine or matters great like overcoming an illness. If you can relate to times like these, then value them. They reflect a pattern frequently found in the scriptures as the passages below show. And, of course, the greatest despairing cry of all, "My God, My God, why have you forsaken me?" came just before the greatest breakthrough of all.

If you are in such a time of difficulty that you cannot feel this message of hope, then, I suggest, simply hold on to what you do have even if it is bitter – and help will come.

Prayer

O God, I am such a shallow creature. I soon despair. I am like a child who throws aside a task at the first hurdle. And I whine. I decide now to endure. I remember your words from St Mark's Gospel, that whoever "stands firm to the end will be saved." I thank you for the fearful symmetry of suffering, endurance and then character. I am awed by the pattern of crucifixion then resurrection. I am frightened to be involved in it. But I accept it. And I dare, foolishly I know, to ask you to etch your death and resurrection more deeply into my life. Amen.

Bible Passages

Genesis 16; Exodus 5:22-23; Acts 18:5-11

Hagar (Genesis), Moses (Exodus) and Paul (Acts) all have times of despair recorded in the Bible; times they wanted to give up. In each case it leads to breakthrough and blessing.

For Meditation

"When my spirit grows faint within me, it is you who know my way!" (Psalm 142:3)

DAY THREE
Pierre and the Vines

"In the day of my trouble I will call to you, for you will answer me"

It was time for my first day of work. The morning was promising. An early bloom of mist lay on the vineyard. It was still cool but the promise of later heat was already to be felt. There was that pregnant calm that portended a hot day to come, even though for the moment one shivered a little.

And there was Pierre. Pierre was in charge of the vines team. I was pleased to note that he was quiet in demeanour, soft spoken. So soft, I struggled with his French. I was both worried and excited by the prospect of actually working in a proper French vineyard. Like so many others I had driven through France in the past and admired the neat rows in the endless fields. I had felt the years of tradition behind the marvellous French wines. Now I was to do a bit of hands-on work. I recalled the wave of envy which had gone around my church when I had announced what I was to be doing. They too had travelled France. I was to become part of this dreamy rural idyll. The first hour was easy enough. We were set to "relever les bras" (lift the branches). We walked along the aisles between the vines stuffing any new or wayward fronds of the vine back within the long wires which ran the whole length of the rows. Occasionally one had to replace the little clips which pulled the wires together between vines. I was surprised to find, that despite the easy nature of the work, I was soon perspiring and my breath was coming in catches. The walk along the rows was clearly further than it seemed. They were very long and they all looked the same. After an hour of this we stopped, got in the battered old minibus and drove to a different field. "Qu'est ce qu'on fait Pierre?" (What are we doing next?), someone asked. "Effeuillage" (cutting off the leaves), he said. There was no great response to this. I didn't know that I had just heard the word that was to be branded into my soul for life.

Effeuillage is simple. Vines in French vineyards are grown to a basic T-shape. The base rises to a height of three feet or so and is then crossed by a bar itself some three feet long. Doubtless they were all trained to this shape by generations of vintners now long gone. From this T sprout the year's new green branches, which will bear the grapes. These grow abundantly and are cropped, I was later to learn, on their tops and sides like hedges. The grapes grow tight into the basic tree at about a height of four feet. The rest of the branches serve only for leaves. It is important to keep the new growth to the bar of the T only and then just to its ends. Growth from the foot of the vines and from the middle of its T is abominated. It offends the French liking for style and neatness. Hence effeuillage, the cutting off of leaves. In modern commercial vineyards effeuillage is achieved by chemical spraying. At La Rebellerie they don't believe in that. "Là, tout est écologique" (there, everything is ecological), that is, they believe instead in natural farming. And that is where mugs like me come in. Instead of chemicals they need people: people who will squat down on the prickly couch grass and clods of baked broken earth, push the overhanging green branches out of their faces and clean up the feet of the vines from the all-pervading and persistent shoots that insist on growing there and on the middle of the T bar. Then they need them to get up to their feet again, walk two or three paces along and do the next one. And then they need them to do the third one. And the fourth. And the fifth. In fact, let's be honest, they need whole teams of people to do nothing else but effeuillage for vine after vine, row after row, hour after hour, day after day.

I enjoyed my first one, I must admit. It was novel. And the second and the third. I think my back started to play up on about the sixth one. I had then been working for perhaps twenty minutes. The row I was working on ran on ahead for many hundreds of yards with hundreds of vines, all needing effeuillage. It was then I think that I realised this was going to kill me. Nor was it going to be a merciful death. It was going to be slow and cruel, and lingering. After an hour every bone and muscle in my body ached. Moreover my hands were raw from "arrachant les herbes" (pulling out the weeds). As a sort of afterthought Pierre had told us to pull out any weeds that were around the feet of the vines too. Well, those weeds were mutants, I swear. Giant sorrels, all knobbly down their stalks. They went through my hands like glasspaper. Walloping thistles, bindweed, and a woody thing I didn't recognise which was the pits to get out. By lunchtime I was screaming inside for mercy, though I knew none would come. Pierre dropped me off at the foyer. I happened to be last out of the minibus.

"Ça va, ce matin?" (How did it go this morning?), he said with a smile.

"Oui, ça va." (Fine, fine).

Idiot, Procter! You should have fallen at his feet and begged for some lighter work. You should have pleaded that you are fat and fifty and soft as butter: that you have a wife and kids, that you would do anything and you mean anything, to get out of effeuillage. As it was, I just gritted my teeth and got on with it. The afternoon was a blur of pain. I simply do not know how those four full hours went by. I do know that at 5.50 p.m., with only ten minutes to go, we finished our rows and stood panting looking at each other. All of us except Pierre that is. He was not panting. He was giving a last loving touch to his vine before looking at us as if we were crazy.

"On commence un autre rang" (We'll begin another row) he said as if there were no alternative, like knocking off a bit early for instance, to start the twenty minute walk back.

So, we started another row, a final backbreaking ten minutes, which I spent devising tortures for the three women in my church who had each separately felt God would do "a beautiful thing" for me among the vines.

Thought for the Day

The trouble was I reckon God was doing a beautiful thing with me among those interminable vine feet. It's amazing how good it can be for you having your world narrowed to whether you can do ten more vines without cracking up. It lets you know how frail your body is. It also lets you know how skin deep is your normal sophistication and poise. Ever so quickly I became a whingeing, column-dodging foot soldier instead of a general.

Try thinking over when God last dumped you in some situation where you were suddenly struggling. When you were reduced to bare essentials in some way. How did you come out of it? Are you now quite glad of it? Did its messiness eventually turn into a beauty of some sort? If so, let us give thanks together.

Prayer

Ah Lord God! It feels like you are forever dumping me in situations where I flounder about, stripped of my usual protections and screaming out for release. Yet even as it's happening, I know somehow that you are doing something authentic, even loving, within me. And I think of Jesus being beaten and stripped and tried and crucified. And that was your love too. So, yes, I accept my hardships and humiliations, thank you for them even. Please help me through them. Amen.

Bible Passages
Psalms 79, 86, 88
All psalms where the psalmist feels dropped in it. Psalms 79 and 86
have elements of breakthrough. Psalm 88 has none.

For Meditation
"In the day of my trouble I will call to you, for you will answer me."
(Psalm 86:7)

DAY FOUR
The Quality Street Tin

"Whoever can be trusted with very little can also be trusted with much"

A big moment at the end of each midday meal was the passing round of the Quality Street box. Where it had come from, I never knew, but after coffee, after cheese, after dessert, after everything else, it was fetched from its place of honour on the chest of drawers and handed round. No decanter of vintage port was ever passed around the Senior Common Room of an Oxbridge college with more ceremony. At my old college (so I was led to believe) it was always the most junior Fellow who had the job of working some drawstring contraption to pull the port decanter round from Fellow to Fellow. At our foyer it was always Michelle who rose from the table unbidden to fetch the sweetie box. At Oxford they presented the port with lots of pretentious twaddle, the dons seemed to need to gild their already over-gilded cage. At our foyer each person's choice was greeted by an outburst of comment and applause. Did someone choose a little square toffee wrapped around with a picture of a rich Dickensian lady? Did someone else choose a long stick-like yellow one? Or a flat disc-like one, also yellow? Or the green coconutty one? Or the strawberry one that looks like a strawberry? Whatever the choice, there was masses of banter and cheering, most of it incomprehensible to me, so colloquial was the french.

When my first turn came, I was quite intimidated by the procedure. I didn't know what to choose and was a little frightened of what response it would provoke. I was constantly being teased all the time. It was good natured, but was having the overall effect of making me not want to stand out more than I needed. However when the packet came my greed overtook me as it always does with Quality Street. I just adore the purple brazilnut and toffee ones. They look so regal with their fine twisted ends to the purple paper, and they taste divine. Deciding to risk the reaction, I delved into the depths of the box and pulled one out. There was an "Aah" of appreciation around the table as if I had selected the finest of wines for the High Table at Oxford and then hoots of laughter for some reason as I unwrapped the thing and put it into my mouth. In the end I was entering into the ritual with as much gusto as anyone else.

As the days went by the level in the box went down. A few days before I was due to go home for my daughter's graduation, it ran out. There was a palpable disappointment. It was oddly childlike. Simple small things had a power to influence the community a lot. Why everyone felt so helpless to replace the packet I don't know. Perhaps it had been a gift and it was not the norm to put Quality Street on the domestic budget. Anyway, there was this flat helpless disappointment, as if we were all children. And into it I spoke. I said that I was going back to England for a few days and that England boasted not just boxes of Quality Street, but whole huge tins of them, and that I personally would ensure that I brought back a large tin four times the size of the now empty box. Applause and cheers rang around the table. It was music to my ears. I had repeatedly felt useless in that place. I never understood what anybody said first time. They always had to repeat themselves and even then I very likely would not get it. I kept doing all the little domestic tasks wrong. I was invariably late for meetings.

It was good to be applauded for doing something really useful. Problem was, I had to get the tin.

"Wot?" said the girl shelf-filler at ASDA, "No, we're not doing tins now. They're seasonal." And she turned away from me.

"Well, might you ask, please? It's important to me."

She swivelled her head round to me without moving her body and fixed me for a moment with weary eyes. Then, "Sha-a-ron!" was yelled past my head like the mistral. If I wore a toupee, it would have been blown off by the force.

"Yeah?" came the reply from a head poked round the distant end of the sweetie aisle.

"We don't do no tinsa sweets this tima year does us?"

"Nah. Seasonal." And the head popped back as quickly as it had come. My helper gave me one last expressionless look and turned back to her shelving. So I bought four boxes, each the same size as the old one. Sainsbury's, Tesco and Safeway were no better and I was going back to France the next day. Somehow it mattered a great deal to provide a big tin of Quality Street rather than four separate boxes. There was some national pride in this and some need to recover my personal pride, which had taken such a denting.

I don't know what made me go into our church office on that last afternoon before my return. I had vowed not to go in there throughout my sabbatical. It's always fatal. I get caught up in parish affairs. But something took me in there, and – you have guessed – there on a table in our church lounge, all on its own, was a big Quality Street tin. I seized upon it like a long-lost brother. It was empty. Even then, I was not out of the wood. Church life is full of booby traps. I am an experienced enough campaigner now to realise that this tin could have been meant to be the centrepiece of someone's children's display, or a vital prop in a play. No matter that it had been carelessly left out in the lounge. Woe betide me if I just took it without checking first. Mind you, I have never previously been free to skip the country after my misdemeanours, as I was this day. Perhaps I would have got away with it. But God does nothing by halves. I checked with Cathy our all-knowing office secretary, who really runs the church. The tin was an empty, disused tin following a recent kids' party, she thought. Since Cathy's thoughts on such matters are as the oracles of God, I was quids in. I took it home and, yes, it was exactly designed to accommodate four boxes' worth of Quality Street. There they lay, after I had poured them in, forming a multi-coloured level all across the top of the tin. Do you know, I think it's things like that Quality Street tin that make me believe in God more than all the doctrines and sermons I have spent so many years absorbing. If I imagine some situation where I had to decide in a split second once and for all if I believed in God or not, if someone had a gun to my head or something, I reckon I would remember that sweetie tin, affirm my faith and die happy.

Thought for the Day

It's the little things in life that are redolent of the big things. I have known someone who gave their whole life to helping the mentally handicapped because of one kiss they received from one sufferer. If you have ever been in love it's probably because of some small irrational thing; a lock of hair, the way somebody ties their shoes. You wonder if all your years of sweat in the Sunday school are worth it, and then a child says something unguarded and you are hooked for another decade. Try searching your life for these "little-big" things. Have you had any? Are you glad of them? Do you want, or need, any more? Prize them. Thank God for them.

Prayer

O God, thank you for these "little-big" things. Thank you for suddenly and strikingly speaking out of very ordinary events to reassure us that you are there. Thank you for training us up in righteousness as we go about life. Please help me to be ever more aware of your good hand upon me and may I prove faithful in small things as well as in big things. Amen.

Bible Passage
Mark 7:24-30
One small saying seems to bring about a great act of healing (29).

For Meditation
"Whoever can be trusted with very little can also be trusted with much." (Luke: 6:10)

DAY FIVE
Guy

"A brother is born for adversity"

Guy was God's gift to me throughout my month. I had only been there one full day – a Friday – when our foyer emptied out. One weekend in four is a weekend off for each foyer. Most members go home for it; any that are left get allocated to another one, except assistants, who hang around and fend for themselves. So, still feeling very strange and disorientated, I found I was to be all alone for my first weekend. I was saved by Guy. He was an assistant at our foyer too and so we teamed up.

Guy was hugely tall and gangly. He could only have been about eighteen. On top of his beanpole frame was a kindly young face. He had been in the foyer all the summer so he knew the ropes and together we cooked and washed up and stuff like that. From the very first he never seemed to chafe with my broken French. He seemed genuinely interested in what I was saying. He took an odd, almost paternal, interest in correcting my French. We went to a photographic exhibition he had seen advertised in the local town. We went to Pierre and Sophie's for Sunday lunch. He turned a desolate time into a fun one.

And he was to be there all my time. We walked the half-mile to work together chatting. We were always together with the others for pétanque (another name for boules, the French form of bowls), Guy being measurer-in-chief in disputed cases. I have an indelible memory of his gangly body; like a male Olive Oil's, coiled in a great spring as he made his throws with the boules.

"J'irai" ("I will go" or, better "My turn"), he would say and then he would in all seriousness adopt a ridiculous pose, his long body like a living question mark, his face stuck forward, before making his throw.

Guy was always kind. He was in the kitchen team. They either peeled onions all day or weeded, by hand, the substantial vegetable gardens. Both sounded terrible and were partly the reason why I stuck to the vines despite everything. At least it was better than the kitchen team. Guy had been doing it all summer, without complaint.

He was hopeless at football, chasing around everywhere like an oversized spider, missing the ball because his legs were so long. He would collapse in giggles at meals at something amusing from his private world. He was deeply devout, thinking maybe of the priesthood but maybe architecture. I just appreciated him. I was very grateful that he was there. At the end of the month I drove him to his home and had lunch with his people. Funny thing was, once there, around the lunch table in their garden, we both reverted to type. I conversed ponderously with his parents and he fooled around with his brother. The bubble of the month had broken.

Thought for the Day

Appreciation. It's good to take the time to appreciate someone, their quirks, their kindnesses, their giving of themselves into life. I often find that once I start dwelling on someone like Guy I unearth much more about them than I had been appreciating. And this is enriching. You might like to try, today, selecting someone from your circle and mulling over all there is to appreciate about them.

Prayer

Lord, please forgive my deep-rooted tendency to dwell on the bad and take the good for granted. Particularly with people. Thank you for the very many good-hearted people who surround me. Slow me down, that I might appreciate them more. Amen.

Bible Passages

Luke 9:28-36
Jesus takes with him especial people up the mountain where he is transfigured.

Matthew 16:13-20
Jesus draws on his appreciation of Peter for an important kingdom-building moment.

Luke 22:1-38
Jesus deeply desires to share the Last Supper with his friends (15) and also gives a glimpse of his especial love for Peter (31-32).

For Meditation

"A friend loves at all times and a brother is born for adversity." (Proverbs 17:17)

DAY SIX
The Serpette

"Do this in remembrance of me"

I am looking at it now as I write. It is sitting there on my desk, next to my computer, which is where it's been ever since I brought it back home, in pride of place. I am not sure of my relationship with it. It is a very crude thing – a worn, wooden handle giving way to a short, curved blade perhaps two inches long. It is a "serpette" (a knife with a curved blade, you can't translate it exactly). It is the basic tool for vinedressers, used to cut off the leaves for effeuillage. I used mine all of every day I worked on the vines. Pierre let me have it for a keepsake. I have just picked it up again and felt its fit in my hand. Immediately, memories flood back almost as if they were channelled through it. There we are, the vines team, sitting in a circle on the grass at "la pause" (the break), the precious fifteen-minute stop we're granted each morning and afternoon. The laughter, the jokes are, most of them, too quick for my French, yet still I feel part of this madcap group. Someone, probably Jean-Xavier, starts a play fight. Four or five will join in. Sometimes I am set upon. I'm put in a headlock or bodily lifted about by three of them. Sometimes it is just a nuisance. I need all my fifteen minutes for rest. Then I snarl and push them off fiercely. I'm getting good at "Arrêtez!" (Stop it!) said with an intimidating rasp.

Sometimes it's fun – stuffing grass down somebody's shirt. And it makes my church diary, full of appointments and policy meetings, seem light years away.

I remember Christine, who brings a full valise of belongings to the vines, discovering she'd lost a trainer. Oh the drama! The tears, the sulky moue of her small face, the wail she set up, the rantings against all and sundry. Then there's Dominic the ordinand quietly restoring it to her. It had got left in the minibus. And then the tears clear away from her face like sunshine after a spring shower.

I remember countless hours bending beside the vines and the growing familiarity with them. I remember the routine of whetting the serpette's blade on a whetstone before each session. By the end I was spitting on the blade and sharpening it up like a veteran, feeling its edge with my thumb. I overdid it once, made it too sharp. Later the blade slipped and cut my finger. It was the forefinger on my left hand. It bled and bled. There was blood everywhere. I was staring at it stupidly when Anna came to my rescue. She took me to the minibus and used the little first-aid kit to patch me up. Even then it still would not stop. It saturated the plaster and the lint and started to run down my hand again. It proved a blessing in disguise. I had to be taken to Roland the doctor at the neighbouring village of Nueil-sur-Layon. He is a member of the community too. It was gorgeous to stop work and relax into the plush of the car's upholstery. It was even more gorgeous to wait in Roland's enormous, cool, flagged kitchen; then to go into his surgery, attached to the house. Roland is an old-fashioned, single-handed village practitioner, such as have long given way to the local health centre in England. He wrapped up my entire finger all along its length with lashings of antiseptic lotion. I wanted that therapy to last all afternoon. I pumped him in my inadequate French about my short, long- and mid-term prognosis. He was very kind and patiently explained. I managed to string him along for a good ten minutes, but what is ten minutes out of four hours?

I remember the sun on the back of my neck. I remember the weirdness of being among the vastness of the vine fields, where your whole world is green and sandy brown but for the tobacco coloured vine feet. I remember passing round the plastic water bottle at "la pause".

I remember, I remember, I remember…

Thought for the Day

Have you got some thing or things which hold memories for you? They could be anything from holiday knick-knacks to important gifts from a loved one. Such things are very powerful aren't they? It is good to go back to them and revisit them. Look at them again. Touch them if appropriate. Probably you have energy still locked up in the memories they hold. Probably love, grief, fondness, regret, happiness are all still lying there latent from the time when you were involved in what you now remember. It is good to tap into your memories fully. Try maybe writing a memoir of some sort. Writing is a useful and powerful tool for recalling forgotten reactions. Apparently the last word spoken by Charles I before stepping onto the scaffold was simply "Remember". And, of course, Jesus in the bread and wine, left us the most potent way of all to remember him.

Prayer

Lord I am amazed at the depth of our power to remember. I am awestruck that everything we have ever experienced is still there locked up in our memories. I think, too, of the complicated defences we use to avoid remembering what is too painful for us. I pray you would prod me, at the end of each day, to remember the many mercies you have shown, and give me grace to face my hidden memories at the right time and place. Amen.

Bible Passage

1 Corinthians 11:23-26

These verses will certainly be familiar. They are used at the heart of the Mass. Note, on reading them today, how much they derive from and call us to the exercise of remembering in depth.

For Meditation

"Do this in remembrance of me." (Luke 22:19)

DAY SEVEN
Les Tournesols
(The Sunflowers)

"See how the lilies of the field grow"

All around La Rebellerie are fields and fields of sunflowers. They are grown as a cash crop. Seen en masse, their great yellow heads are like so many comic figures – clowns or flowerpot men. But, the longer you look at them the less comic they become. Their faces, comprised of their large grey-brown seeds, are heavy with portent. It seems surprising that they can hold them up to the sun at all. They seem weighed down with grave matters, the burden of their own fruitfulness. Yet, of course, they can and do hold up those massive heads. Not only hold them up but turn them to follow the sun on its travels through those wide open West-of-France skies. And here is where their personae change yet again, and they become like children. Children who, in innocent selfishness, simply want to get the best for themselves and drink in the best of the sun all day long. They have no politeness or inhibitions as adults might. They are plain enough to have no shame in taking what they want. And no harm is done because there is plenty of what they want available. Lots of sunshine to go around. They can just bathe in the elemental rays of the sun all day long. They are prevented by their place in creation from fighting one another and so the farmyard selfishness of childhood is excluded.

Here's a poem I wrote about them:

> At first, they grin a ninny grin
> And hang their heads.
> The yellow of their petals
> Yokels' straw-hair.
> Tall and gawky,
> With wide, vacant faces
> And nothing to say.
> A field full of them,
> Toothless and silent.
> You, passing in your tourist car,
> Think it charming,
> If a little rural,
> In all conscience.
> On impulse, you stop,
> Get out and walk across.
>
>
> From close.
> Each face,
> Looming over you
> Becomes an insect eye,
> Huge and many-prismed
> And each prism a seed,
> A sandy-grey pyramid,
> Ancient of ancestry,
> Latent of oil,

Able, each one, to propagate
A thousand more like itself.
And its plant to you is suddenly
Fecund and fearful and tall
Greater, quieter, stronger than you
And your metal box.

Then, as you move away,
In no small fear, wondering
You make, as you feel you must,
One last look back
Over your shoulder
And see
Neither peasants nor timeless gods
But children.
Stood together
Innocently, greedily, gently
Jostling to get the light, the warm
Of the Sun
Into themselves.
Unashamed, unaware
Of aught but him and them
Needing nothing
Of travel and sophistication.

Thought for the Day

Pick one of the three personae of the sunflower I offer you: whether it's
the gawky clown or the grave thinker or the child. Dwell a little further
on this choice. Why do you think you made it? Is it a choice made from
habit – the kind you would normally expect to make, or is it a choice
made from something else? Weigh up your motives. Did you find it

easy to make your choice? Did you care? Do you associate yourself with the persona you chose? If yes, do you like your association, and why? Decide whether there is anything to learn about yourself as you relate to your choice, and to the sunflowers themselves. And, perhaps, decide to look at flowers generally more closely. Apparently when Jesus says "Look at the lilies of the field" it is a strong command – "Look closely and deeply until you get the meaning."

Prayer

Lord thank you for the complexity of our make-up. Thank you that we can be more than one thing at once, yet still be one person. Please help me to explore more just who I am and how I relate to all you have made. And please help me to take due time pondering on these things until I receive your intended meaning. Amen.

Bible Passages
1 Corinthians 1:18-25 *on being a clown.*
Proverbs 8:1-36 *on being full of heavenly wisdom.*
Matthew 19:13-15 *on being a child.*

For Meditation
"See how the lilies of the field grow." (Matthew 6:28). The word for "see" is strong. It means "dwell upon until you get the meaning" or "drink in significantly".

DAY EIGHT
French Cuisine

"I have eagerly desired to eat this Passover with you"

A month on a French farm! As someone who likes his food, you can imagine how I was looking forward to the meals. I had been hoping for a combination of the bulk of food you associate with farm meals and the quality of cooking you associate with France. But I had reckoned without one or two things. My first challenge was eating every course off the same plate. You ate your salad. Then you ate your meat, often on its own. Then you ate your vegetables. Then your cheese and biscuits. Then you ate your fruit salad, or fool or whatever dessert, each new course being served on top of the remains of the one before, onto the same plate. Being able to see the remnants of mayonnaise and the sauce the meat was cooked in through the otherwise fine syrup in which the fruit salad had been served was off-putting for me. Then there was a similar economy with glasses. The same glass served for your water, then for the welcome and regular inch or two of wine, then for black coffee with a sugar lump. It was good news when you were on washing up duty as I was to discover. But it turned my usually strong stomach.

Next was the cuisine itself. Not so haute. I ate a lot of burgers, usually more than half raw. There was lots of powdered instant potato as well, often over-watery. Haricot beans, boiled into the water, as a course on their own, were a bit grim too. Well, I can tell I'm breaking your heart, so I'll move on to pleasanter things.

Breakfast was good, but you had to be quick. Overnight our highly sophisticated cafetière had, in obedience to its microchipped insides, produced some glorious coffee. The problem was, if you were not in the dining room within a minute of the morning bell, you didn't get any coffee. This was because Philippe had arrived and siphoned off a good pint's worth into his vast breakfast bowl. Then Jean-Benoit had done the same. And that was it. My first morning, strolling into a delicious aroma of pure ground coffee, I was imagining the heaven of a mug of it with my croissants. But I was appalled to find the pot was empty. Philippe and Jean-Benoit were busy slopping their bread in it and slurping up a full bowl's worth, tipped directly into their mouths. I was left to make shift with some weak cocoa stuff. Ever after that, you need not worry, I was out of my oratoire like a greyhound as soon as the bell went. All I wanted was a nice mug full and I made sure I got it.

And I did get some of the excellent French meals I craved. There was one splendid "pique-nique deluxe" (super picnic) with salmon and oysters and melon and olives and pâté and glorious fleshy tomatoes, halved and stuffed with rice salad, and whole shrimps and Roquefort and Camembert and wonderful crusty baguettes with masses of butter. And there was another outdoor barbecue where we had fabulous long sausages as well as a wonderful array of "tartes" – tartes aux pommes, aux poires, aux citrons, aux pêches (apple tarts, pear tarts, lemon tarts, peach tarts) – and simply stacks of crêpes (pancakes) with maple syrup or crushed bananas or sugar and lemon added to taste. All washed down with the whites and reds of the vineyard itself, and eaten under the trees shaded from the wide summer sun of the French West.

I don't know if this affects you very much. As I say, I'm not much bothered about food myself. I just thought you might be interested.

Thought for the Day

Reflect on what you eat and try to relate it to how you walk with God. "There are those who live to eat and those who eat to live." Which are you? "What you eat is what you are." Do you find that is true of you? Do you crave food? Or can you take it or leave it? When under stress, do you eat more or less food? And when do you eat? Often? Or rarely? In a hurry mostly? Or at leisure? And with whom do you eat? Your partner? The children? Or are you mostly alone? And where do you eat? At a table? Off a tray? Do you say grace? If so, is it before or after the meal – or both? Reflect a little on all these things. What do you think God makes of your eating patterns? Imagine him sharing your food with you. What would that experience be like? A privilege? An embarrassment? What can be learned from this?

Prayer

Lord, thank you for food. Thank you for all the varieties and combinations and versatility of the foodstuffs in the world. The vigour of the way you have made growing things is almost frightening. I am sorry for when my appetite gets depraved – for being greedy, in short. Please forgive me. And please make me eat in awareness that so many people go hungry. Amen.

Bible Passages
Daniel 1:3-16
Daniel refuses to defile himself with the king's food and wine.

Jeremiah 52:31-34
The exiled king Jehoiachim dines regularly with the king of Babylon.

For Meditation
"I have eagerly desired to eat this Passover with you." (Luke 22:15)

DAY NINE

Pardon my French

"And having been warned in a dream not to go back to Herod, they returned to their country by another route"

It quickly became all too apparent that my French was not good. In my interview with Dorothée, who looks after the assistants, I could see her waiting for the halting words to fall from my mouth with painful anticipation on her face. She assured me that a number of assistants come who can hardly speak the language either but that they soon got by. There was one other English person there when I arrived, a student finishing a gap year. An engineer. He was fluently laughing and joking all around. I know he had been there some months but it didn't help. I had to ask people to repeat themselves nearly all the time. When it came to my turn to say anything, finding the phrases was hard and what I did say came out mechanically. I was limited anyway to banalities because my French was so elementary. So much in conversation stems from putting a little originality or irony into the thing. The members of the community with learning difficulties often completely baffled me. I understood many of them no better at the end of my stay than at the beginning. In the vines someone would say something and it would be meaningless. Then they would repeat it and still I would look blank. I could see my stock dropping dramatically. Guillaume once gave the archetypal Gallic shrug and turned away contemptuously, leaving me there. And, once, when I was asked to read grace at the meal, which I did in my best 'A' level oral exam accent, Espérence, our House Leader, put her head in her hands in amused despair, just saying softly, half to herself, "Aah, l'accent!" (Oh, that accent!)

All this was the more galling because I fancied myself at French. I had got the French prize at school. On holidays I had enjoyed cutting a dash in shops and restaurants doing the ordering and mostly getting it right. I had been to a refresher class at night school in preparation for my month and been the star pupil. Now here I was tongue-tied and de-skilled. The other assistants, youngsters less than half my age, were multi-lingual. Agathe was Polish with fluent German and French; Christina was Italian, living in Paris, with fluent French and Spanish; Guy had German and Spanish, whereas I could not follow above a third of what went on at meetings. I took to pretending I had understood, often nodding and saying "Oui, d'accord" (Yes, OK) when I had not the faintest idea what had been said. When Espérence told us her grandmother had just died I failed to understand, and also missed the subdued atmosphere it created. I buttonholed her about something pettily domestic straight after the meal at which she had announced it. She bore it well but it was crass of me. A family came to dinner one evening, former community members, still living close by. I followed hardly a word. I think what saved me from being blanked out all together were the other forms of communication. I worked hard, didn't shirk. I enjoyed the knockabout – the playfighting and other teasing. I laughed alongside them, pantomiming and fooling, as with the Quality Street. Games were good levellers, especially the ritual evening pétanque (French bowls). When Espérence once commanded, for some reason, a late-evening, open-air swimming party where some were reluctant to brave the cold, I led the way in and splashed about. All this said things. It said what was true – that I meant business about being there, that I wanted to be part of the work and life of the place. And they took me on board. I think, if I had been able to speak more fluently, I would have tried less hard in these other respects, and that would have been a loss of something important.

Thought for the Day

Is the direct route to something you need being blocked right now, in the way my involvement in the community was hindered by the language barrier? Are you stymied in some way about anything or anybody? Do you keep bumping up against barriers whenever you attempt something? Maybe you are being asked to explore alternative ways of approach. And maybe those ways – like my having to rely on deeds, not words – might be more powerful than those you would ordinarily use. Think of someone you might describe as a "closed book". Or of a situation you regard as a "closed door". Dwell on them somewhat. Allow God to stir ideas for other approaches within you. Perhaps it's okay to leave well alone for now. But perhaps he is suggesting a different way which could be of benefit all round. Think about it.

Prayer

Lord, I come before you to try and take some time to think about … (fill in your particular situation).You know how stuck I have been with it all. Do you want me to do anything different? And if so, what? I am going to take the next five minutes (that's a long time for me remember) to stay here and be open to your ideas. Amen.

Bible Passages

Joshua 6

God gives some very unusual battle plans for the destruction of Jericho.

2 Samuel 5:17-25

David consults God twice. The first time God's direction is to act in a straightforward way, but the next time it's more roundabout.

Ezekiel 3:25-26

Ezekiel has the power of speech taken from him. He then has to do his prophecying through acting (see chapters 4 & 5).

For Meditation

Of the Wise Men: "And having been warned in a dream not to go back to Herod, they returned to their country by another route."
(Matthew 2:12)

DAY TEN
Pétanque

"I tell you the truth, unless you change and become like little children, you will never enter the kingdom of heaven"

Each evening after the meal Paul would stick his face right into mine and with a rubbery grin, ask, "Pétanque, Père André?" (A game of boules, Fr Andrew?)

In case you don't know pétanque is boules, a version of bowls but played with metal balls and on gravel not grass. It's a big national pastime in France. Out we would go to the pea shingle in front of the foyer. Paul would be like a dancing bear clanging the metal boules together and jumping up and down in excitement. Guy would be there too, incredibly gangly. The young student girl volunteers, Agathe, Christina and Anna all played with a fierce will to win. Anne-Marie, one of the staff, would come sometimes and fool about. And Philippe would sit on the bench and brood and boast of his days as a champion in Provence where the boules were half as big again.

Here I learned for the first time how to play properly. To begin, two shots were taken at the cochonnet (the "piglet", or the jack as we would say), one from each team. Whichever team was furthest away was obliged to keep shooting until they had either achieved a nearer boule to the cochonnet than their opponents or run out of boules. Thereafter the other team had their goes. Various scenarios were possible. Sometimes it was very tit-for-tat, as the game see-sawed this way and that. At other times your opponent got in a good boule close to the cochonnet and proved impossible to dislodge. Then you usually lost all your boules in succession trying, to no avail, to get inside the good one from your opponents and had to stand helplessly by while they gleefully heaped up more points against you as they had their goes. Sometimes you had this sadistic pleasure yourself but not as often as having to suffer it, it seemed.

There were hot disputes about whose boule was nearest. These were settled by a variety of ingenious measuring devices. Different people would totter one foot in front of the other, tightrope-style, from their boule and then reckon how far up their trainer the cochonnet came on their final step. Guy would get on his hands and knees and move his long spatulate hands spider-like over the distance, counting the spans. Sticks, purses, mobile phones, kitchen knives were all given work as makeshift measuring rods. For some reason we never got organised by having a ruler or even a piece of string. Probably we sensed that would spoil the craziness of it all.

You play first to fifteen, scoring one point for every boule you have nearer to the cochonnet than your opponents. Some were quick games – with, say, four a side and two boules each you could score up to eight a time if you were lucky. Some took until it was growing dark and Espérence emerged like my mum of old to warn it was getting on for bedtime. And, truly, we were like children in those evenings. Whether it was the young girls, not much more than children to me, screwing up their pretty faces with fierce concentration and then leaping with excitement if they did well; or Guy, all arms and legs, here, there and everywhere throwing, measuring, announcing the score; or Paul cavorting like a bear; or Philippe sitting waiting to go last, his blue eyes like chips of ice, trying to mask his delight at winning with a "don't care" manner. We had the seriousness of children at play too. It was our whole world to try our best to win for forty minutes or so. And then, when it was over, it was forgotten. I can still hear the particular crunching sound of the metal boules as they hit the gravel in my memory. It evokes for me a feeling of well-fed ease after the day's hard work, cigar smoke on the evening air and bonhomie.

Thought for the Day

Think a little. When did you last play a game? Of anything. What was it? Cards? Badminton? Scrabble? Do you play games often? Or rarely? Or never? And – what do you do in the evenings? Do you spend enough time being childlike? Do you play enough? When last did something trivial enthral you? It's an amazing tonic. It has something to do, I think, with becoming like a child in order to get in touch again with something important and innocent. Remember Jesus' words of guidance and warning: "Unless you change and become like little children, you will never enter the kingdom of heaven" (Matthew 18:3). Notice the need to *change*. There needs to be some definite move made – playing more pétanque, I reckon.

Prayer

O God, please forgive me for filling my life with dull, adult, pressing matters. Help me relax. Help me opt for something pointless. Help me meet others in the magical world of fun and games. Help me be a child again and so may your kingdom come and your will be done in me. Amen.

Bible Passages
Mark 9:33-37; Matthew 18:1-9
Both are passages where Jesus teaches the value of childlikeness.

For Meditation
"I tell you the truth, unless you change and become like little children, you will never enter the kingdom of heaven." (Matthew 18:3)

DAY ELEVEN
The Scouts

"He went away sad"

One night we couldn't play pétanque. We had to go to the scouts' campfire and sing songs, explained Paul. It took a little time for me to get his drift. For one thing I didn't know we had any scouts around. True there had been some extra young people at our meals. But all kinds of people seemed to come and go at La Rebellerie and I had taken little notice. For another, the French pronounce scouts as "scoots" and scouting as "scootisme". It sounded so odd that I could not understand. Once I did understand, I was miffed. I liked our games of pétanque. And I had bad memories of scout campfires myself. What was it again, that daft song we sang ad nauseam when I was a scout? Ah, yes, "Ging gang gooly, gooly, gooly, wotcher, ging gang goo. Ging gang goo." (Repeat) Hailer. Hailer-shailer. Hailer-shailer. Hailer-Hoo."

I mean, really, to sit about as an adolescent and be made to sing baby talk like that did me damage I reckon. I recall grown men coming out of their tents with their "camp blankets". These were ordinary blankets festooned with all kinds of naff badges. Place badges from previous camps; Whitby, Llanberis and so on. Badges of other far-flung outposts of scouting; Zanzibar and Indonesia, got presumably by mail-order since no one travelled that far in those days. I don't know what other kinds of badges. I just know there were lots of them. And they sat in these things and sang Hailer-Hoo.

So I told Paul I was not fussed about the campfire, nor the scouts, and spent a solitary evening smoking and pretending I was enjoying myself but really I was lonely. When they all got back obviously having had a good time, I just went off grumpily to bed.

But then I kept meeting the scouts. We went round the zoo, some of us that Saturday, and bumped into all six of them in uniform. They were really pleasant youngsters. They showed up again at meals and were fun. The following Monday morning, I discovered they had been assigned to our vines team. They worked hard. I was with a comely, demure girl who was a pleasure to work and converse with. (I was fit enough now to be able to talk and work at the same time.) She cut François down to size too. François was one the assistants, a student from Paris; a tall, handsome womaniser who had collected a harem. He didn't like work and was good at finding soft jobs for himself. This particular morning he came along as "official photographer", gliding around taking snaps. He found this combined laziness and flirting very well. After he had hung around us rather too long, Charlotte, I think her name was, straightened up from bending to a vine foot and said with delightful false sympathy, and a nod at his camera, "Ce n'est pas trop dur, cela?" (It's not too difficult, your work?)

And she made big, contemptuous eyes at him. His smile froze on his face and he loped off. I liked that. We shared a grin, and got on. The other scouts were great with the team. There was one girl scout who teased all the regulars to death. She was full of fun, yet she had an underlying respect for their neediness, you could see that. I got a break from being wrestled around too, which was good.

And then on their last morning, at morning prayers, they presented a really very lovely piece of wood sculpture with a Calvaire (Calvary), which they had made for the worship table. So, in the end, I had to change my mind about the scouts and "scoutisme".

Thought for the Day

Have you ever lost out by turning something down out of sheer negativity? You have received an invitation to something and you would really quite like to go, but you are foiled by a reservoir of miserable unwillingness to put yourself at risk. It could be a dance, or dinner out, or a service of worship or a long weekend. It matters not. But you simply don't allow yourself to do it because you are some sort of jailer to yourself. You have decided you don't deserve such things. Or you have a bad history with it, like me and scouting. Or, worst of all, you have got yourself in a generally miserable permanent state where you screen out all sorts of good possibilities on an ongoing basis. Today's a day to cast around. See if there's something good you could and should get involved in. And do it.

Prayer

Lord. Have mercy. Please have mercy. And do not destroy me, as I deserve. For I am a wretch who turns down your kind offers of life, again and again. For no better reason than plain misery. I bury my one talent. It is fear. It is defiance. It is selfish. It is a refusal to share myself with others and with you. Thank you that you forgive. And (here goes another kamikaze prayer) please send me soon a challenging opportunity to get involved somewhere and to ditch my negativity. Amen.

Bible Passages
Numbers 14
The people refuse to enter the Promised Land out of fear (see Hebrews 4 for a commentary on this.)

Matthew 25:14-30
The parable of the talents.

For Meditation

Of the rich young man after refusing Jesus: "He went away sad."
(Mark 10:22)

DAY TWELVE
The Stars

"Is not God in the heights of heaven? And see how lofty are the highest stars!"

I could not sleep – a not uncommon thing for me. So I got up and went out into the warm night air. This involved no more than stepping over the low threshold of my bedroom window and thence out onto the gravelled frontage of the foyer. Once there I looked up in wonder. The sky was alive with stars. Trillions of them. There was the great badger stripe of the Milky Way right down the middle like a rough swipe with a paintbrush. There was the Plough in a space of its own. I followed the line through its two end stars and found the North Star, less isolated but somehow brighter than its neighbours. I found Orion, or rather his three-star belt. Then, having exhausted my impoverished stock of astronomy, I just stood, my head tilted right back and gaped. A profound stillness held all, yet I was aware of the life of these countless stars and galaxies as full of a boundless energy which dwarfed the very earth on which I dwelt by more multiples than mathematics could cope with. It was hard to imagine these vast systems turning in wheels of galaxies, each of which were travelling at unimaginable speeds and over distances I could never make my mind comprehend. It was hard to stop myself treating them all as a nice nocturnal wallpaper that God had put up from some rather upmarket, celestial B&Q, much as a parent might put up Paddington Bear wallpaper for a child. Was I right to try and force myself to think big and adult in this way? Perhaps it was better to subside and let myself reckon that God had made all of this as no more than a backdrop to human life. I recalled senior preachers of the evangelical world, at some august and godly gathering, opining that there is just us in all creation. Us and God. Oh, and of course the angels. I remembered how ludicrous I thought that view then. How British and self-centred and assured. I can see, now, their chins stuck out and their nods of assent around the room. The idiotic brass neck of it! Only them and their conventions in all the vastness of the universe, with the angels as sort of spiritual valets. The blinkeredness of it. Yet, perversely, maybe they were right. It was better to let these mighty things wash over one, to take them as a wastrel God's great bounty and get on with life.

I moved round to the paddock next to the house to avoid the intrusion of the house's night-lights. It was even stiller here – and darker. How peopled the heavens were that night! Was it only imagination or was there some faint far, far distant song being sung, the tune to which these mighty engines moved in their great dance? And how light they seemed, these twinkling pinpoints, which in reality were massively heavier than anything I might contemplate. And how neighbourly, when in truth we were separated by every division of space and time and form in quantities so vast as to defeat even thought about them. More than neighbourly. There was kinship. Those things up there were my fellow creatures. The same hands that had formed my clay had put them together too in all their might. The same one who had given me my two feet and hair, sweat glands and grey eyes had formed these Lords of Matter. And, if the New Testament is to be believed, he had been pleased to dwell as one of me. Amazing.

I realised I had grown cold. Time to go in. How long had I been there? No more than thirty minutes. It was all I could take. How long had they been there? Aeons. Aeons my wallpaper. Aeons, the humour of God. With myself his infinitesimal clown.

Thought for the Day

Well – when did you last spend time looking at the night sky? Is it perhaps time to do it again? Especially if it's near Christmas when our wonder of the stars fits in with the Christian tradition. Spend time stargazing. And let your thoughts free-wheel through the heavens, as do the great stars themselves. You will not go unrewarded.

Prayer

Great, great God. Great, great Lord. To whom the stars may be no more than playthings for all we know, look upon us your frail children in love and mercy. We worship you for your great might, but also we dare to believe you have planted the stars in us. We see them in the fragrant heads of our children. In acts of love, often amid squalour. We see them in the burning flame of faith, tracking through our history as do Pleiades and Orion in the heavens. Please be patient, you to whom the ages are as nothing, and bring us and the stars to the new heaven and the new earth. Amen.

Bible Passages

Isaiah 40:25-26; Job 38:31-33
These are both passages where God asks us to dwell on the majesty of the stars and on the majesty of the one who made them.

For Meditation

"Star differs from star in splendour." (1 Corinthians 15:41)

"Is not God in the heights of heaven? And see how lofty are the highest stars!" (Job 22:12)

"He also made the stars." (Genesis 1:16)

DAY THIRTEEN
Anne-Marie

"Do not judge, or you too will be judged"

One day at the table, when I returned from the fields, there was this odd person. She was short, stout and pasty white in complexion. I approached her to shake hands and give a welcome, only to receive much voluble French which I took to mean "back off". It did mean just that, I later learned, but not because she didn't like me. Rather she had some illness, which made it better to avoid human touch. I bracketed her at the time, I'm afraid to say, as one of the needy, insecure types whom the foyer took as guests from time to time over and above the routine of caring for those with learning difficulties. The next morning I was a little puzzled to see her hanging out of an upstairs window down at the centre of the little hamlet that is La Rebellerie in noisy conversation with some others.

Then a few days went by, after which I had more or less forgotten her. That evening though, Espérence, our regular guardian, needed to be away, and who should come to replace her but Anne-Marie, as I discovered her to be called. Apparently she had recovered from her mysterious illness. She greeted all with double kisses on both cheeks and joined in the pétanque immediately and with aplomb. She turned out to have a great gift of humour. She adopted a ludicrous posture on one leg for her turns to throw, which broke up the rather severe atmosphere Philippe was creating by his determination to win. She proved to have great way with Yves, one of the most distant and mysterious of community members. Yves always seemed so sad and worried. He turned out for work like a dapper businessman, neat and tidy. He spoke in a breathy, deep voice which seemed to come from another world. You had the sense that he lived in a way that only loosely connected with ours. Sometimes at the foyer I would sense him having private thoughts of his own, whether laughter or despair I could not tell. Every night at bedtime, whoever was there, he would walk into the lounge, alarm clock in hand, and check it with the clock on the wall. Then he would leave. You felt he would do that even if the place were on fire. I rarely saw him laugh. Anne-Marie would fix him with her eyes and emit a weird kind of animal call to him, full of fun, and his head, often bent, would lift and he would laugh. He had the most open of laughs it transpired, childlike in its vulnerability. His solemn face would split and his gappy teeth would show in a grin of complicity with her. They would exchange these noises for a while, Yves giving forth great guffaws of laughter. She told me later that he was very worried about getting his things packed properly for the coming holidays which were not far away. How she knew this beat me, for Yves scarcely spoke, but she had a deep understanding of him and of the other community members.

Anne-Marie was a great teller of set-piece jokes. Her version of the wide-mouthed frog was delightful. Perhaps it tells better in French but I reckon it was Anne-Marie's rolling eyes and infectious sense of the ridiculous that made us all laugh like drains at the punch line. Tongue twisters, too, were a speciality: "Combien sont ces six saucissons? Ces six saucissons sont six sous." (How much are these six sausages? These six sausages are six sous – a small French coin.) Try saying that a few times with Anne-Marie's funny, pink face all agog at you, challenging you not to break down helplessly with laughter.

Her birthday fell while I was there. In her honour we had the "pique-nique deluxe" (super picnic) that I have already described. Each of us had a plateful of the most delicious combination of food. Towards the end someone called attention to her feet, which were bare. This was rather tactless, I thought, because her toes were all out of line and some were webbed. At this Anne-Marie immediately stuck them into the very middle of the picnic cloth and began a great discourse on how her feet were the product of a distinctive ancestry unique in all France. Only she and her forefathers had the like. They demonstrated her ancient lineage deep in the historic nobility of the nation. To this day I have no idea if she was serious. I thought again how free of spirit she seemed and generous in her self-giving to all in the group.

I discovered she had been at the community for some fourteen years. Far from being the perhaps inadequate person I had first thought, she was one of the mainstays of the place. She was at that time fixing up everybody's summer holidays. We got chatting about it before the guests arrived for one of the barbeques. She made no show of it but it sounded a delicate, detailed job requiring due regard to the different levels of disability among community members. I realised again how far wide of the mark my first impressions had been.

Thought for the Day

Think of someone you know whom you initially misjudged. Someone who has turned out very different from your first impression of them. Has this change been for better or for worse? If, as with me and Anne-Marie, it has been for the better, take a little time to give thanks for that person. For their richness. For your debt to them. Think how you might have lost all that wealth if you had avoided them because of your first impression. If it turned out for the worse, perhaps it is important not to lose whatever was the first attraction. It is probably still valid. And maybe resolve, if you are still in contact with them, to understand what has made them disappoint you.

Prayer

O Lord, forgive us judging so. We do it all the time. Slotting people into categories, measuring them by our small standards, jumping to conclusions. Of course we are the greatest losers in this, missing so much good in so many people. Please help us to take our time with people, to expect the best, to encourage, to remember you have blessed all your children with great inner resources, and that we all bear the mark of Jesus somewhere. Amen.

Bible Passages

John 1:43-50

Nathanael almost misses out by jumping to conclusions from his first information about Jesus. In response Jesus overcomes any initial hostility and Nathanael becomes a disciple.

Mark 8:22-26

The blind man's first vision is incomplete, Jesus takes him through a second stage and his sight becomes whole.

For Meditation

"Do not judge, or you too will be judged." (Matthew 7:1)

DAY FOURTEEN
Pierre and the Rain

"When you pass through the waters,
I will be with you"

As I have already said, much of my fate at La Rebellerie lay in Pierre's hands. For eight hours a day Pierre owned me. A word from him could set me to unbroken backbreaking monotony or to something more tolerable. It depended on Pierre whether I was to scrabble around interminably in the unforgiving clods of broken earth around the vine feet, sweat dripping off my nose-end, hands sore, my back killing me. Or whether I was to get away with something lighter, like lifting the odd branches that had fallen out of their wires. Every morning at eight I waited for the critical moment when Pierre would pronounce on the day's work. He always spoke lightly as if it were no great matter. He did not seem to know that his words either condemned me to a grim day's endurance test or left me with the hope it would at least be bearable. Pierre was slight of build, softly spoken, with huge roughened hands. He always had a gentle demeanour and an eye for how people were. But the vines came first. There was an inner core of the fanatic to him. I have described already how, on my first day, with just ten minutes to go, Pierre had ordered us all to start another long row of vines, apparently totally unaware of our bedraggled, exhausted state. He himself had looked exactly the same as at eight in the morning. Finally and at long last, the minute hand of my watch crawled up to the hour. Christine said in a kind of defiant croak, "C'est six heures", (It's six o'clock) and slung her big bag over a shoulder. Pierre was opposite me. He looked up at this, and then at his own watch. I could sense he didn't want to believe it was time. He whipped off a couple of runners from his vine and lovingly ran his hands down the gnarled stump. Then he stood up. "Bien," he said again, "On part" (OK, we'll go), though you could tell it was a wrench for him.

Imagine then, if you will, my feelings the first morning it rained. It was the following week. Perhaps I had by then become a little hardened to the work, perhaps I hadn't. I had been chatting to Dominic over the weekend. He was a fellow volunteer who had been there all summer. I had mentioned Pierre's fanaticism to him. He confirmed it by explaining how a fortnight before it had poured down with rain for two days. I can still hear him saying "des grandes averses" (huge showers). Yet Pierre nonetheless had them all out there in the open fields all day, both days. I recalled that rain and those showers. They were when I had been travelling down. Very wet it had been. My mind did not want to contemplate what it would be like to do all that repetitive harsh work getting thoroughly soaked in relentless rain all the long day. And then to have to do it again the next day and even the day after that.

But there we were. It was once again the fateful eight o'clock in the morning. As usual we stood under the roof of the big Dutch barn grouped around Pierre, waiting for his directions. There would be no arguing, whatever they were. The rain simply poured down. It drummed on the roof. Rivulets were coursing along the driveway outside. I recall a couple of the office ladies arriving in their hatchbacks and running into the buildings under umbrellas. Hervé stood erect and impervious to all this.

"Bien," (Good) he said, as crisply as ever, the piercing eye looking out on the day. In that moment I despaired. It was the fields for us for sure.

"Il y a trop de pluie, je crois. On restera ici en épluchant des piquets." ("It's raining too hard, I guess. We will stay here and épluche some piquets.")

I looked across at Dominic who shrugged, surprised. I did not know what piquets were nor what you did to épluche them but we were going to be dry and that was good enough for me.

Thought for the Day

Reprieves. Have you had many? Times when you expected the worst only, and often at the last minute, to discover yourself let off the hook. Cast your mind back through your recent life or maybe you will need to go back further and recall the last time you experienced a reprieve. Was it a big matter? Or something smaller? Relive it a little. How did it come about? Who had you to thank for it? Try to relate it to the fact that all of us owe our salvation to the greatest reprieve of all, the forgiveness of our sins by Jesus Christ.

Prayer

Lord, thank you for life's ups and downs. Thank you even for nervousness and the sense of being outfaced at times by life's challenges. Thank you for often stepping into our lives by way of reprieves – though do you have to leave it so late so often? And, of course, thank you for forgiving us our sins. Amen.

Bible Passages

Genesis 22:1-19

In this famous passage, God gives Abraham (and Isaac!) a last minute reprieve.

Matthew 18:23-35

This parable is about God's reprieve for us and ours for others.

For Meditation

"When you pass through the waters, I will be with you; and when you pass through the rivers, they will not sweep over you." (Isaiah 43:2)

DAY FIFTEEN
Épluching the Piquets
(Peeling the Stakes)

"I'm going out to fish"

As I said yesterday, I had no idea what it was to "épluche" nor what "piquets" were. It turned out that éplucher is French for "to peel" and piquets are "stakes" – wooden stakes. About every twenty feet or so along the lines of vines is a wooden stake about four feet tall. There must be thousands of them at La Rebellerie's fields alone. The wires, which run all along the vine rows, are fastened to them. The stakes and the wires between them create a framework to hold the vines' foliage in place, by exactly the same principle that a domestic gardener will create a frame for tomato or runner bean plants. Over time these stakes rot and need replacing. With huge numbers of them in use all the time this creates a permanent need for new ones to replace rotten ones. The new ones are made, it transpired, from fir tree trunks. Without thinking much about it I had walked past the large stockpile of these trunks that stood near the main farm buildings on my way to and from work every day. We were now about to spend a day turning trunks into stakes.

No sooner had the word fallen from Pierre's lips than the more senior of the team's members disappeared off up the yard to reappear a little later driving tractors with several tree trunks lying across their forklifts at the back. Meanwhile we lesser folk had gone off to get some scimitar-shaped tools I had not seen before. They were the exact shape of hand scythes but with two handles. I was still vague about how they were to be of any use to us, but I was soon to be enlightened. Guillaume and Vincent had pretty quickly offloaded some twenty or thirty tree trunks from their tractors. These were, on average, about eight feet tall and a foot in diameter, though they varied quite a bit. Félicien and Jean-Xavier set about splitting them and then we were each given a quartered tree trunk to lean against one of the metal pillars that held the barn roof up. The scimitar, scythe-shaped things were used to peel off the bark. You started at the top, worked the blade of the thing under the bark and then ran it downwards. It was very satisfying. The bark was, on the whole, amenable to being peeled off in this way. It came off in long strips, leaving a satisfying stretch of bare white wood. It was very like stripping wallpaper. Sometimes you came across a more recalcitrant bit of trunk, but it usually yielded to some extra effort and was all the more pleasing for the challenge. True, it was quite tiring to have to keep lifting your arms above your head to reach the top places, but this was a small price to pay for the gratifying and absorbing nature of the work.

By way of change from this épluching, there was always the option of a go at splitting the trunks. Now, for once I could bring some background expertise to bear here. At home, I keep our large open fire stocked with logs and am a dab hand at splitting big pieces of timber, sometimes with a wedge and sledge hammer. I had not split whole trunks this way, I must admit, but I easily made the adaptation. To belt a couple of wedges into a length of timber and feel it split into two neat halves along its grain is deeply satisfying to the soul. In both the peeling and the splitting were all sorts of tiny variations and trials of skill. Could you split in one blow or should you, more judiciously, take two? Could you peel efficiently round a funny nodule in the wood?

And so on. Add to this the customary badinage and informal competitiveness within our team, the facility for stopping and having a smoke pretty often, the frequent passing of the secretaries which made me feel macho as I wielded my axe, and you can see how the day passed in happy preoccupation. I was as absorbed in it as a child. And all day it was pouring down with rain. Sheets of it rippling down until the driveway formed big channels and the drumming on the roof almost drowned out conversation. And I was dry and happy and not out in those shelterless fields getting soaked.

By the end of the day the tractor team had taken away loads of peeled and split trunks (for some reason we did not saw them in two then and there, nor did I ever find out the necessity of peeling the bark.) And a large pile was left. This pile stayed out under the barn for the rest of my stay, and every time I passed it my heart always warmed with satisfaction.

Thought for the Day

What simple tasks are there which you like doing? I like stripping wallpaper and splitting logs. My wife loves washing and ironing (thank goodness). What is it with you? Cooking? Mopping floors? Laying carpets? Making bread? Washing the car? Make a list for yourself. Try not to omit anything. Now – thank God for them. They are his gifts. Incidentally, probably you feel not a little bashful about the enjoyment you find in them. But resist this. The fun and the absorption and the simplicity they afford keep you childlike. We thought of the value of play in this regard earlier. Try now dwelling on the value of simple, absorbing jobs in helping you be restfully recreative and absorbed in what you are doing. It's surprising, too, how to switch off and do some simple unthinking task can allow the mind to freewheel, so that we come out of the wallpapering or whatever with problems solved or some new avenue of creative thought begun.

Prayer

Lord, thank you for rhythm and restfulness in life. Thank you for the balance of our bodies and our minds. Please help me to make sure my life includes the right amount of easy work which is restful for my over-busy mind and which gives me good exercise.

Bible Passage

John 21:1-19

Here Peter, after all the stress of Jesus' death and amid the uncertainty of understanding his resurrection, impulsively chooses to go back to something familiar, and more physical than mental. It leads him to a great revelation of the risen Christ and a vital conversation with him.

For Meditation

"I'm going out to fish." (John 21:3)

DAY SIXTEEN
Espérence

"Unless a kernel of wheat falls to the ground and dies, it remains only a single seed. But if it dies, it produces many seeds"

On my first day at La Rebellerie, after I had arrived and been given lunch, they took me to our foyer or "household". It was called La Croisée and it lay a quarter-mile from the central buildings, on its own save for Pierre's house. I have already described its creamy walls and red tiled roof. It lay drenched in sun. I was told that Espérence, who was in charge of our foyer, would see to me soon. She did not seem to be around at the time. Perhaps she was sleeping. So I took a seat under the trees opposite and wrote a letter home. I had just finished it when she came out across the gravel to greet me. I'm afraid I was lost from the moment I saw her. I just had a blurred impression of a mass of chestnut hair, shorts, a sleeveless T-shirt, sandals and deep, deep hazelnut eyes. She had been speaking to me in voluble French, I realised, for some moments with me just staring at her, mouth open no doubt, hearing not a word."Pardon?" I said, with a shrug. It means sorry in French. She repeated it all again, an amused look of surprise at how dumb I was coming into those eyes. She was to find me exceedingly dumb all month because every time she spoke things seemed to swim around in my world. It was hard enough to get people's drift first time anyway in French but with her I had to contend with her beauty. And so there was always that puzzled look behind the eyes which I took to mean something like, "He looks intelligent. They said he was a priest of some experience – why is he such a geek?"

This effect was added to by the fact that I kept doing everything wrong around the place. I committed innumerable small domestic sins. For example, I put the glasses back in the wrong place; I didn't twig at first how the washing up rota worked and missed my turn (cruel this because I often washed up voluntarily); I asked, casually, if I might have a drink from one of the bottles of aperitifs standing temptingly in the kitchen. This provoked consternation because apparently we only drank them on certain special occasions; and I put my washing in the washing machine wrong and then hung it out in the wrong place. All these things invoked tellings off from Espérence. These were embarrassing for me as she was no more than half my age. I was angry at such humiliations, being used to giving orders not taking them. Anyway, I have always chafed at the multitudinous offences it seems possible to commit all the time in household life, wherever I am. They also seemed to matter a lot to Espérence. There wasn't too much humour or sense of proportion, it seemed to me. I suppose in community life matters of order count for more.

Overall, Espérence seemed somewhat scratchy. She wasn't around much except to do the necessary at meals. She was substituted for by Anne-Marie and Sophie, Pierre's wife, several times. After a couple of weeks she announced that her grandmother had died and she would be away for some days. I guess that lay behind it all. Of course, I missed the drift when she told us all. The critical word "décédé" (deceased) in

French eluded me on first hearing. I think it is used in preference to "mort" (dead) which is regarded as harsh.

In the second half of the month she became more outgoing. She organised Anne-Marie's birthday "pique-nique deluxe" (super picnic) which I have mentioned before. She fixed up a swimming party for everybody which went well, but she looked tired about the eyes. I gathered that she was shortly to leave the community. It made me ponder on the dedication and cost of being a community leader. Whilst, outwardly, the life of our little household seemed to potter on harmlessly enough, there must have been innumerable concerns involved in it. There were issues of medication, of liaison with families and social services. There were meals, rotas, shopping, washing, bathing details, all constantly in play. And, most of all, I guess, there would be the endless interplay of personalities, both established community members and birds of passage like me, who needed instruction. I was not surprised to learn that they get through house-leaders pretty quickly at L'Arche.

Thought for the Day

Dedication. What is there to which I am dedicated? For what am I happy to put up with much tiresome drudgery because I believe in the outcome? My family? My job? Anything else? What is costing me anything? It's worth the effort of examining this from time to time. If there's nothing, then, nearly certainly, I am impoverished. We need that which is greater than ourselves, if we are truly to find ourselves, whether that's a war or a baby. If we feel, on the other hand, swamped by our responsibilities to the point of having no life of our own – and this I suspect is the more frequent thing – then maybe we need to prune something out of our lives. Or maybe we need to die, in a sense, for the greater cause.

Prayer

Lord Jesus Christ, help us know when and where you are calling us to be crucified alongside you. Help us avoid self-inflicted martyrdom where you don't want it. But, more, help us take up our cross and follow you when we should. Amen.

Bible Passages

Mark 8:34-38; Mark 10:32-34; John 12:20-26

These are all passages where Jesus teaches of the need to find life through death, the gaining of life through losing it.

For Meditation

"Unless a kernel of wheat falls to the ground and dies, it remains only a single seed. But if it dies, it produces many seeds." (John 12:24)

DAY SEVENTEEN
Dignity at Work

"Indeed there are those who are last who will be first, and first who will be last"

"André!" (Andrew!) I looked up somewhat taken by surprise at the call of my name. I had been busy for a while with my vine feet. There were long stretches of solitude as one worked. The caller was Félicien. He was standing hands on hips some yards back up my row, looking at me askance.

"Il faut arracher les herbes" (You must pull up the weeds) he said with impatience, pointing as he did to a clump of sorrel I had overlooked. Those clumps were the pits. They certainly were very different from the gentle little green sorrels I pluck from my garden beds so easily. These were massive with long strands of rust-coloured flowers that seemed to strip the skin from your hands as you yanked at them. They gripped the concrete-like earth too. I had probably had a go at this one and decided to leave it be for once. This was not good enough for Félicien obviously. I suppose I could have bridled at his telling me off like this: he was not in charge of me. Pierre was in charge and he rarely dressed people down like this. I could have brushed him off. There was nothing he could have done about it. But I didn't. I trotted back shamefacedly to the spot and I squatted down obediently at his feet and struggled with that sorrel under his supervising gaze until it came out.

Later, having ample time to muse over the incident, I found myself smiling at the irony of the middle-aged, Oxford-background clergyman being treated like a naughty schoolboy by a young man of twenty. I decided the reason I had accepted it was most probably the earnestness Félicien had shown. It had really mattered to him, that sorrel, and the keeping neat of those endless vine rows. His work and his dignity were bound up in it. I thought of Guillaume, another serious worker. He was busy some rows away driving a tractor with wide arm attachments trimming the vines. It looked like it took some skill to keep the arms from flailing and to drive the tractor so it kept them aligned correctly. I thought of his deep concentration when we had once had a talk on wine production, during which my attention had been all over the place. I reckon you are close to at least one of the great contributions of L'Arche when you see young men like these, who would have been on the employment rubbish heap in open society, doing real work – work that needs doing, which holds its place in a competitive economy, which they can do better than unskilled types like me. L'Arche has given the Féliciens and Guillaumes and many like them the dignity of mattering and being seen (to themselves as well as to others) to matter.

Thought for the Day

Well, you have probably just had it. But, take it a little further. There was me, a man accorded much respect in his work, being stripped of his dignity for a bit – and it was good, for me and for life. And there were Félicien and Guillaume enlarged by being accorded dignity in their work. There is much tacit indignity for people in their workplaces. Working under fears of redundancy, scrabbling for promotions, people being moved about as if they had no families or communities. How is it for you? Are you compromised in any of these ways? Or, conversely, would it do you good, like me, to be pulled down a peg or two? Or three?

Prayer

Father, the forces of economics seem so massive and impersonal. They dwarf us. It's hard to feel that you are the Lord of the workplace too. Help me in my work. Help me fight for justice where I should. Help me know the when and the where of how to change if I should. Humble me (get the dose right here Lord whatever you do) if I could do with it. Where I hold responsibility for others, help me uphold their dignity. Amen.

Bible Passages
Luke 14:7-11; Matthew 20:1-16
Both are about the last being first, and the Matthew passage has lessons about the workplace.

Amos 8:1-14
For God's judgement on unfair economic practice.

For Meditation
"Indeed there are those who are last who will be first, and first who will be last." (Luke 13:30)

DAY EIGHTEEN
Being Ignored

"If anything is excellent or praiseworthy — think about such things"

It was a glorious day and a lovely scene. The occasion was the annual Friends of La Croisée barbecue. We had set up trestle tables under the two trees outside the foyer on the grass. I had had the job of supervising this and very lively it had been. Getting them level had been enough of an exercise. My team of Paul, Yves and Michelle proved to be very biddable but a bit over eager and my every command to move a table along a bit or sideways a bit had been turned into moving it a yard or so, which had meant starting all over again. Anyway we had got them in position at last.

The real fun was covering them with the paper banqueting roll. There was a slight breeze. Not such as you would notice were you not dealing with ten-foot lengths of flimsy paper outdoors. The fun we had with that stuff! I would station Paul at one end with the furled roll. Michelle was at the other end waiting for it. Yves was our roller in chief. I was on hand for emergencies. Yves would begin to roll. The idea was that

Paul would keep his end held down as Yves rolled, that Yves too would keep his spare hand flat to the table and that Michelle would collect her end, cut it with the splendidly large office scissors and we would sellotape it all down. I could intervene at any time to help out. Fail-safe and simple, as have been all the many plans I have made in this life. My problem is, as I have told a troubled world many times, that nobody listens properly to my instructions. If they did, there would be world peace. There was not world peace at La Croisée that sunny morning. That little breeze played lots of games with us. It played let's-get-lots-of-white-paper-stuck-up-in-the-trees. It played let's-wrap-Yves-up-like-an-Egyptian-mummy. It played let's-get-Procter-over-excited-so-he-interferes-and-tears-the-paper. It played let's-let-them-finally-get-it-flat-down-and-nearly-sellotaped-and-then-whip-it away-again. Lastly it played let's-get-them-all-helpless-with-laughter-and-then-fetch-Espérence-out-to-give-them-a-royal-telling-off.

Even when we had got those tables ultimately covered having used a year's supply of roll and sellotape we still had to negotiate things like interleaving paper plates with paper serviettes and setting out the paper cups. No messing now. Espérence, much distracted in the kitchen catering for thirty people, was on the warpath. We used so many pebbles to weigh things down the tables looked like Chessil beach. I was fearful as to what she would make of this but I think she got past caring.

However, these troubles, as St Paul so rightly says, were not worth comparing to the glory that was to be revealed. Before long the scene had become a festive country idyll. We sat or stood in the sunshine under those trees, glasses in hand. The tables were spread with all manner of foods. I especially remember the salads and the tartes-aux-pommes (apple tarts). Both were done as only they can be in Western France. But there were pâtés, quiches, pastas, meats. There were crêpes, gateaux, and gorgeous fruit. There was cream, there was wine. Our white table covers were hardly visible. Naturally bonhomie was everywhere. The children were prized, especially Aimee, Pierre and Sophie's seven-year-old, who has learning difficulties herself. Later there was to be pétanque of course but also football in the field next door. This was much enlivened by thistle patches, a one-in-four slope and a transformed Espérence now chasing everywhere in high spirits uttering a frequent, earthy "merde!" when she missed the ball. There was also Claudette, Pierre's old donkey, to be negotiated. She was especially useful when forming "the wall" at free kicks. Sideways on, she was bigger than the goal.

Yet my memory of all this is spoilt by one little thing. There was a man there who ignored me. I didn't notice at first in the general mixing, but as time passed, it became inescapable. He adeptly dodged away whenever I hove into view. Whereas most of the visiting "friends" took some interest in me as older and a bit different from the usual student-type assistants, he was plainly avoiding me. I nailed him in the end, of course. I can't have people ignoring me. He minimised the conversation and moved off. His behaviour puzzled me. I didn't smell, at least not until after the football. I was usually an OK bloke. What was the matter? Then it dawned. It was my poor French. He didn't want to be bothered with the effort of conversing so brokenly. I was sure of it. Sure because, I realised uncomfortably, I had done the same to overseas guests myself often enough. Well now I knew what it was like. It was shaming. And alienating. And infuriating. It cast a shadow over the sun. Nor was it my fault. Or was it? I couldn't tell. And it made me think – what is it like for those with learning difficulties? I thought of Ben in my own church, who goes around everyone during coffee-time after the service, shaking hands. And we all shake his hand back with a smile and then get on with our "real" conversations. And off he wanders again. Do he and others like him feel a smarting sense of rejection whenever they're in company?

Thought for the Day

For a start: do you, like me, often let one bad thing spoil a whole lot of good? Do you dwell on the one bad thing in the day, sucking at it like a lozenge, forgetting all the good? If so, do work on reversing it. At the end of the day, free-float your memory until it picks the best thing about the day. Then suck on it. Draw all the good you can from it. You will be surprised at the depth of that little blessing no matter how small it seemed. In Ignatian spirituality, it is called the "examen of conscience", and very good for us it is.

Second: who do you avoid? Pick just one. And think why you do it. You are probably not alone in doing it. Probably most people avoid them. Do you need to do something about it?

Prayer

Lord. Thank you for all the good you send. There's loads. Even on bad days and in hard times. Help me dwell on it and draw from it all the goodness wrapped up even in small parcels. I suspect there are unlikely places where you send goodness too. Help me see the goodness wrapped up in people I am, at the moment, avoiding. Help me get past that which is putting me off. Amen.

Bible Passage
Philippians 4:8-9
This passage is full of positive thinking. It is worth learning by heart.

For Meditation
"If anything is excellent or praiseworthy – think about such things." (Philippians 4:8)

90

DAY NINETEEN
A Slice of Life

"Be content with what you have"

The timetable at La Rebellerie ran a little earlier than I am used to. Bed was at 9.30 p.m. Breakfast at 6.30 a.m. The rising bell at 6 a.m. Often enough I was awake by 5 a.m. these summer mornings.

Every other day, I would go running. I found it quite something to be stepping over the threshold of my bedroom window and out into the grey quiet morning at that hour. It was usually still misty. The vine leaves were damp with dew. It was light but the sun would not be up yet. It's always a lurch to start running. My body rebels every time. But once I get going, I hit a rhythm. I would leave behind me the big ugly concrete water tower that dominates our skyline and head for the delicate grey church tower at Clercy-sur-Layon on the other side of the valley. As it neared, the beauty of these western French villages enchanted me all over again. Muted stone buildings seeming almost extensions of the landscape, decked with the neatest of trailing geraniums. A "mairie" (town hall) complete with tricolour, even for this tiny hamlet of a few hundred souls. The village centre, an irregularly shaped space for parking surrounded by plane trees. The light grey church, a confection of stone rising to the cone of its thin spire. You might expect it to be blown away by the breeze. And the faded brown façade of the boulangerie (bakery)-cum-village bar – quiet as the grave this early morning. On arrival up the hill I would stop, panting like a horse, and pace around the car park, hands on hips, head drooped. Then I would head back. All the little landmarks of my journey: the bridge over the river, the turning for Nueil, the next-door field of vines, the Calvary at the turning for La Rebellerie proper, finally, the big phallus of the water tower and home. Then the blessed relief of stopping and the glow of self-satisfaction running around my limbs like liquor.

Then there would be a shower, stooping low to avoid banging my head on the bathroom's sloping roof and holding the shower nozzle above my head. There was no lock on the door and Anne-Marie, another early riser, came in once and found me naked. There was little embarrassment; she just gave a snort and went out.

Later cross-legged, trying to meditate in my oratoire-cum-bedroom, blessedly free of flies in the mornings, I would breathe deeply and happily. Much was well in my life. Nay – all, all is well. And all manner of things shall be well.

Thought for the Day

Take a slice of your day. Any slice. Could be your early morning routine like mine, or some other. Lunch (if it exists). The early evening. Then go through it slowly in your imagination. Maybe write it up into a narrative. Maybe, even, express it in some other form – a poem, a picture, a sculpture, a flower arrangement. Dwell on your thoughts or work. What has it aroused? Wellbeing, as with me that morning? Or maybe something darker. Despair? Anger? Whatever it is you have delved into how things truly are for you. Hold on to that and return to it later. You may be thereby able to know you are happy, underneath it all. Or that you must change something.

Prayer

Forgive me, Lord, for always skimming the surface of my life. For gobbling down your kindly daily meals, complaining to you as I cram my mouth that they aren't enough, that I starve. Help me go gentler. Help me savour your unfailing gifts each new day. Help me drink my cup in life to the full. Amen.

Bible Passages

Philippians 4:10-13; Timothy 6:6-10; Hebrews 13:5

These passages are about true contentment.

For Meditation

"Be content with what you have." (Hebrews 13:5)

DAY TWENTY
The Knee-brace

"It is better for you to enter life crippled than to have two feet and be thrown into hell"

After a couple of days at the vines Pierre noticed my struggles. He came up to me carrying some odd contraption in his hand which looked at first sight like a calliper for a lame leg. He offered it to me and explained that it was a proper vine-worker's knee-brace. You could strap it on and when you got down on one knee to tend your vine it gave a pad for your knee to rest on. Also a little seat for your bottom came up somehow, so that the weight of your body was borne.

It seemed a good idea. I warmed to the feeling of using an authentic French device of this sort. I strapped it on. It was certainly different. As Pierre had said, it saved one's knees the rough contact with the soil every time and it was fun to subside onto the little seat. After some time though it began to rub my knees every bit as much as the ground had done, chafing the skin. And somehow it threw my balance as I knelt. I felt all lopsided. It was awkward to walk about too with it strapped on.

But that wasn't truly why I dispensed with it in a couple of hours or so. It was pride. I thought the others were looking sidelong at me. I sensed their pity and very slight contempt for me in needing the thing. It wasn't much. They were kindly enough but I thought it was there. At break or when we had a huddle at the end of a completed vine-row I felt different. Just walking up to the group was different because I was walking with the shackling knee-brace on. To be crude, I felt a cripple. Not able to take my medicine of hard work in the vine-field. So I took it off. Rather, for me, to do my back in (this was a real possibility – I had slipped a disc the summer before) than occupy the role of weakling. I would rather have the sweat of a day's intense labour than show any need to be cosseted.

Thought for the Day

Would you have done the same? To my mind there was good and bad in what I did. Good, in the grittiness, the determination, the if-they-can-do-it-so-can-I. Bad in the pride, the need to feel self-sufficient, the need to keep up with the crowd. There was also something deep going on, a blend of the good and the bad, some life-preserving herd instinct that drove me on. Maybe you find yourself in some pressure situation where it is hard to keep up. Maybe you need to sift your motives a bit to find out what part of yourself to go with. And maybe it's best to bring it all before God, trying to discover what he thinks about it all.

Prayer

Dear Lord, thanks for the challenges – I suppose. Life would be dull indeed without them. You do tend to overdo it somewhat though, you know. Have you ever thought of easing back on the throttle? No? What? Time is short and the battle hard? Yes. Yes indeed, Lord. And you it was who bore the brunt of it. And still do for that matter. So be it. Help us then to fight within and without, to know your mind and to win the day over our rebel emotions. Amen.

Bible Passage
James 1:2-7
Which both tells us to rejoice in our trials (2) and to seek God's wisdom in them (5).

For Meditation
"It is better for you to enter life crippled than to have two feet and be thrown into hell." (Mark 9:45)

DAY TWENTY-ONE
Gerhard

"Seek peace and pursue it"

About halfway through my time at La Rebellerie, there appeared on the scene Gerhard. I don't know where he had been the first fortnight, perhaps on holiday. He was German. He had blond hair and blue eyes. He was tall, lean and, somehow, other-wordly. A gentle and earnest chap. Yet, in some way, difficult to describe – he was different from the rest of us. We all wore the oddest assortment of clothes for work. There were football shirts, T-shirts, shorts, jeans, overalls. Yves always turned out dapper as if for a day's tourism rather than the sweat of the vines. Gerhard's collared shirts and khaki shorts and white sun hat were that bit different, but also had an indefinable air of isolation. It was as if he had come from another age or clime. He was Pierre's deputy, having served nearly a year at the community. He worked us just as hard. His French was quick and he kept on top of the slight shirking and the horseplay that always went on with us. He once, blessedly, sent me off to do some work with my trenching tool all on my own for a morning in a particularly overgrown part of the vineyard. I loved that solitude. I just needed it at that time, an unexpected island of peace amid the teamwork. I don't think Gerhard did it out of a sense of my psychological needs of the moment. It was for the sake of the job, but it was the kind of light, happy chance I somehow associated with him. He unfailingly used the knee-protecting contraption which I had been too proud to use even though I could have done with it. And it seemed no mark of shame on him, as I felt it would have on me. Gerhard was different. He wore a neckerchief of green with spots on it, which made him look curiously old-fashioned. He was a head taller than the rest of us with crinkly hair cut unusually.

I talked with him at some length once. He was leaving that summer to go and study mediation and peace-making at college in Brittany. I could feel that he had, from deep down in his soul, a sense of the world where it was not just wrong but deeply abnormal and absurd for people to be at conflict. He was protestant, the son of a Lutheran pastor and he did not attend the community Masses, nor Mass at the local parish church on Sundays. He lived out of the community too – in a room in the nearby village of Nueil-Sur-Layon.

We had a team trip out near the end of my month, which was also the end of the community's year. The barbecue was a bit slow to get the sausages cooked and we took to singing for entertainment, mainly childish or bawdy songs I fear. At a pause in proceedings, Gerhard, unprompted, stood straight upright and sang, solo, a most beautiful ballad in German. At any rate it sounded like a ballad. I suppose it too could have been rude, but I doubt it with Gerhard. We all clapped him. He had done a Gerhard on us – ennobled us, sweetened us, come to us from an altogether lighter, better place of being.

At the big farewell ceremony at the year end, they gave Gerhard a gift case of the community's wines. Not something I would have wanted myself in his shoes, having slaved over the vines for a year. He took it, not so much graciously, as distantly. It mattered little to him, the wine or gifts at all, or all the work. He made a short, gracious speech. He had passed through us without ever truly being of us and yet he had blessed us profoundly.

Thought for the Day

Take someone you know who is eccentric. Dwell on your feelings about them. What are they? Are they on the whole negative – such as revulsion, distaste, irritation? Or more positive – such as interest, refreshment, fascination? Puzzle over why that person is eccentric. Try to think through where they are coming from in life. Try to analyse where you are coming from with them. Probe to find out if any avoidance of them is more truly an avoidance of life itself, for they share life with you. What can you do to celebrate more deeply those who don't fit "normality"?

Prayer

Lord, it is the enemy who would have us all the same and you who made us all so different. Forgive me the fear which makes me put so much of my energy into being sufficiently like the others that they will accept me, and then tries to be that little bit better than them. Help me relate first to you, frightening though that is, and then to others. Help me please also to celebrate variety in a conformist world. Amen.

Bible Passages

Genesis 14:18-20; Hebrews 7:15-17
Melchizedek is someone who occurs in the Bible unannounced and unexplained, yet appears to be an important pointer to Christ.

Joshua 5:13-15
Here Joshua meets a mysterious person called "the commander of the Lord's army" to whom he pays reverence.

For Meditation
Thinking of Gerhard's calling to mediation:
"...do good; seek peace and pursue it." (Psalm 34:14)

DAY TWENTY-TWO

In Charge

"Blessed are the poor in spirit, for theirs is the kingdom of heaven"

Before long I was in charge of the vines team – strictly on an acting basis you understand. It was not that I was anything special at the work. It was that Pierre seemed to have a lot of other things to attend to and Gerhard, his deputy, had a penchant for splitting us up into smaller units. We assistants were a bit like junior officers or school prefects. In the absence of higher authority, we were supposed to take charge. It was all a bit tricky. You had to keep your troops together for one thing. People worked at different speeds. They also sensed that they were off the leash for a bit with just a rookie like me in charge so they played up. Félicien and Jean-Xavier stopped for too many fags and chats. Philippe and Vincent started to play fight. Christine took to complaining rather. It could get difficult.

One sunny morning, when I was in charge, Jean-Benoit went flop-bot on me. He slumped down like a recalcitrant camel and would not budge. There is a very gentle regime in La Rebellerie. You cannot use threats or the other nefarious means that I have used on recalcitrant teenagers at house parties in my time. You can but cajole. Successful cajoling, I now discovered, depends upon clever use of just the right tone of voice and the right phrase. This is very difficult in a foreign language. I found I could not shift him. My team were getting far on ahead up the vine rows by now, their shirts just dots of colour against the all-pervading green. So I left him and went back to sort out my other workers who themselves were up to all sorts of shenanigans. It proved a very trying morning. I was back and forth up and down those stifling rows of leaves between Jean-Benoit and the rest of the gang. I once got him to his feet but he only walked a few paces with me and then flopped down again. I began to have more sympathy with police at demonstrations dealing with sit-downers. I was in a cold sweat as to what Pierre would think of all this when he found out. I don't know how it would have ended if Gerhard had not turned up, for my team were ever farther from Jean-Benoit and I was running about like a demented hen. But he came an hour before lunch and took Jean-Benoit away with him. Apparently this was not his first flop-in and there was a way to deal with him.

Certainly, at lunch, he was back to his old self. He had a way of saying your name in an odd arresting tone and then a snippet of English he had learned. It went something like, "Inndiroo! 'Ow are you? Inndiroo! 'Ow are you? Inndiroo! 'Ow are you?" And then,"I really lerve you!"

He had a store of silly sayings into which he inserted your name. I found it okay normally, but frazzled from my fraught morning, to see him sitting there bright-eyed and bushy-tailed taking the wotsit out of me, when he had caused all the trouble, was a bit strong.

After lunch there was Mass. I went to the loo beforehand to avoid having to cross my legs throughout. As I got there Jean-Benoit was just coming out. He gave his hyena's cackle, "Inndiroo! 'Ow are you? I lerve you!" and went on his way. When I got in the cubicle, he had not flushed it and it stank. I rested my head on the wall. I had had enough just now of Jean-Benoit.

Half an hour later I entered the lovely, homely community chapel. There was the altar, specially decorated with flowers. There were large candles already burning. Christine was clanging the bell for dear life. And there, robed in white, seated with Bertrand (who had also given me a difficult morning) ready to serve the priest, was Jean-Benoit.

They had such coy expressions on their faces. I find it hard to recapture the exact mix. They were still naughty boys all right. They were feeling privileged. They were a little nervous. But, for me, a saintly light came from them. There was something deeply right about the two of them being robed in white up in the sanctuary, while I was in the body of the church in working clothes. I rejoiced in the justice and love of God. Truly these two "poor in spirit" as some might think (Matthew 5:3) were nearer to God than me. And I must strive to be like them, not the other way around.

Thought for the Day

I hope what you have just read makes you thoughtful! To apply it a little more, try searching around among your acquaintances for someone whom you despise or annoys you, if only sometimes. Dwell on them. Pray for them a little. Bless them. Does this release any secret blessings they may have for you? Does it affect the light in which you see them? Perhaps, as with me and Jean-Benoit, you shrink somewhat and they increase in value.

Prayer

Lord, those Beatitudes are tough. Are you sure you got them dead right? I spend my life trying not to be poor in spirit and you are telling me I've got it wrong. I guess in fact what I do is spend my life running away from the fact that I am poor in spirit. And you are telling me to face up to it – and that then I might see you clearer. Yes. Okay. It's still hard though. I do love you, you know. Amen.

Bible Passage
Matthew 5:3-12
These are the Beatitudes, a collection of sayings at the beginning of the Sermon on the Mount which "turned the world upside down." (Acts 17:6, RSV translation)

For Meditation
"Blessed are the poor in spirit, for theirs is the kingdom of heaven." (Matthew 5:3)

DAY TWENTY-THREE

Mass

"Forgive and you will be forgiven"

There were two types of Mass at La Rebellerie. There was Sunday Mass at the local parish church along at Nueil-sur-Layon and there were the community Masses in the chapel on site. The ones in church were an education for me, as I had not attended a typical French Roman Catholic Mass before. I was surprised how many people were there for one thing. I had been hearing dire things about French Roman Catholicism: only six priests were ordained in the entire country the year before my stay, the average age of serving priests being seventy-two, attendance figures plummeting. But, here we were in a deeply rural setting and the place was fairly full. The numbers were no doubt augmented by the presence of our nearby L'Arche community but there were still plenty of people there other than us. I enjoyed discovering the format of the worship too. The priest gave the homily and, of course, presided at the Mass proper. But the rest; music, prayers and the liturgy of the word, was led by lay people who had plainly put in much thoughtful preparation beforehand. The overall impression was one of a calm, shared experience. I found it nourishing.

The community Masses were similarly thought out. Members of the community had prepared readings, prayers, and bits of drama. The cool of the chapel was itself a benison after my hot, sweaty day in the fields. The low beams of twisted wood in the ceiling gave deep succour on their own. It was amusing to see fellow team members with whom I had been clowning and play wrestling only an hour before, now like sombre schoolchildren delivering their part in proceedings. The old priest who had come along to celebrate Mass was obviously respected and spoke of a recent trip to Eastern Europe where God had been moving among the poor people. I sat on my bench, crammed in between I know not who, and breathed deeply of the peace and simple beauty of it all.

Then it was time to file forward for the bread and the wine. As I queued up I took my cue from Sally, another English assistant who had been here before. She crossed her arms over her chest and bowed for a blessing instead of receiving the bread. As a non-Catholic she could not receive. Nor could I. So when it came to my turn I did the same. I was not prepared for my reaction. As I bent forward and the priest blessed me, needles of painful tears hit the back of my eyes. Some mix of anger and baffled love welled up in my gut. It was an effort to get back to my place in the po-faced manner which for some reason, is often deemed appropriate to such proceedings. When I sat down my ears pounded and my breath came in spurts. I was angry. I was hurt. I was surprised. I felt excluded. I had put in nearly a month among these people. I had come to feel they were my family in some way. Had I got it wrong? I knew of course that there was no question of my being consciously excluded. I was used enough to the anomalies of Christendom, the artificialities of denomination. As a priest I know about the historical and doctrinal divides that are in play and have reckoned to respect them. Still, I could not get away from the hurt. I was surprised by it. I so loved these people and had learned so much about God from them. How hard not to be able to share the sacrament as one of them. How it stung.

Thought for the Day

Kicks in the teeth come hard, particularly when you have been especially soft in your approach. How to deal with them? Understanding and forgiveness. We must try to understand where the kick has come from and why it has been given. Probably the kicker hardly guessed at the effect of their action. And even when the hurt was consciously or recklessly given we must forgive – just let it go. Maybe we should voice our hurt in an attempt to create understanding and a better situation, though, in my experience, it often misfires. It's all so, so hard, but it's the only way.

Prayer

Lord, I can hear you. It's okay. "You must forgive your brother, from your heart." This and much more. I know there's no messing with it. I just find it difficult that's all. So please help me. Help me to let things go. Help me to minimise the wrongs done to me and maximise the good. Amen.

Bible Passages
Luke 6:27-42; Matthew 18:15-35; Luke 7:36-50
All these passages are about forgiveness and loving those with whom we are offended.

For Meditation
"Forgive, and you will be forgiven." (Luke 6:37)

DAY TWENTY-FOUR
The Sandal

"Wear sandals but not an extra tunic"

I was given a sandal as a parting gift for my sabbatical by a parishioner. It was not a full-size one, but a miniature one, on a leather thong, to be worn around the neck. I wore it day and night throughout my month among the vines.

She, my parishioner, had bought the sandal in Assisi on a visit to the shrine of St Francis. I have always admired the Franciscan ideals. Among them, for Franciscan friars at least, is the commitment only to wear the simple Franciscan brown robe and a pair of sandals. Simplicity of clothing was important to Francis. He had been the son of a wealthy cloth merchant who had bitterly resented Francis's conversion to an active Christianity and had threatened to cut him off from the family clothing fortune if he persisted with it. In reply, so the story goes, St Francis stripped off all his clothes then and there and, from then on, only wore the single rough brown robe characteristic of his order. The summer before I went to France, I had myself walked the Yorkshire dales for a month, clothed only in a Franciscan-style robe and carrying no money. It had been a marvellous experience, if a little hairy at times. So my sandal was a reminder of that and of the espousal of simplicity at L'Arche.

L'Arche's ideals are also marvellous. Jean Vanier, the founder of L'Arche, has written widely on how he came to begin the movement and how, for him, it enshrines seeing the power and beauty of God in weakness and vulnerability. When you are wearing an open-toed sandal you are vulnerable. You can be stamped on. You can't run very fast away from trouble. You can't stamp your feet in noisy anger or a military march. This, perhaps, parallels the situation of people with learning disabilities, who do not, often, enjoy the defences cultivated so carefully by people without such disabilities. That is why I wore my sandal, to appreciate this.

Of course, as you will probably have thought by now, feet in sandals are marvellously free. They can breathe. They do not get cramped. They can feel the earth they walk on much more sensitively. They experience much less stress and weariness than shod feet. And they don't stink. So it is at L'Arche. There among all in the community, amid all the disadvantage, I sensed a rare and innocent freedom. There was a strange peace around. There was freedom from pretence. There was no competition or self-vaunting – no stink in other words.

Thought for the Day

Play an imagination game. Start by imagining you are wearing jackboots or some other heavy footwear. Let your imagination work on how you walk in them. Do you march, stamp, scramble or what? And how do you feel? Powerful? Protected? Perhaps encumbered? Then change. Imagine taking them off. And putting on open sandals. Now imagine walking around in them. Compare your feelings with being booted. What do you feel now? Which do you prefer? Finally, what sort of footwear does your soul walk in habitually? Are you in need of any changes?

112

Prayer

Lord save me from all unfeelingness. Even if I have to go barefoot through life, slow and hobbling like the pilgrims of old. Even if I have to look silly and risk being trodden on. If it takes that to keep me in touch – then it's okay. Amen.
P.S. I must be mad, because I bet you will take me up on this.

Bible Passage
Mark 6:6-13
Jesus sends out his followers in poverty; vulnerable and dependent on others.

For Meditation
"Wear sandals but not an extra tunic" (Mark 6:9), and
"Nor can foot feel being shod" (from *God's Grandeur* by Gerard Manley Hopkins)

DAY TWENTY-FIVE
The Photo

"If I just touch his clothes, I will be healed"

My time at L'Arche was beginning to draw to a close. Whether it had passed quickly or slowly is hard to say. As I have described in these pages, there were times when it was torturously slow, yet, alongside this, was the impression that my whole month was just one all-too-short moment of beauty, one glimpse of heaven, over tantalisingly soon, almost before I had realised it had begun.

On the Wednesday of my final week, we had a vines team day out. At the morning community meeting of that we day we caused much merriment, arrayed as we were in our smart casuals rather than the usual working togs. Guillaume looked like James Dean in tight black jeans and shirt. With his serious face and smouldering, ice-chip eyes he made a very different figure from his habitual boiler suit. We climbed into our minibus not, as usual, to trundle out to the fields, but to go to the "Musée du Vin et des Vignes" (Museum of Wine and Vineyards) in a neighbouring town. After that we visited a working vineyard close by, particularly to inspect vines whose leaves had been burnt off by a machine at the height where the grape bunches grow in order to let the sun ripen the bunches more effectively. I watched the faces of my fellow workers as they listened to the man at the musée and to the local grower. They were full of interest. They asked all manner of questions. They pulled at their chins doubtfully as they spoke with the grower over whether the expensive burning procedure was worth it. I thought again of the gift of worth and dignity L'Arche had given them, placing them thus on a level footing with this prosperous, professional man. No – not given, for surely the gift of worth and intrinsic dignity is every person's birthright from God. Not given then, but restored. Given back, where an uncaring world had seen it taken from them, regarding these precious, precious people as some sort of drag on a productive society.

Lunch was yet another barbecue. We were hungry by then and the food rather slow to get cooked. Horseplay began and not always so good-natured. I found myself suddenly rather tired and hoped not to get put in a headlock or bodily lifted up or any such thing. But soon we were fed and watered and things settled down.

Then it was farewells. They thanked Gerhard. Then they thanked us, the assistants. And they had something for us. It was a photo of the vines team. I remembered, now, its being taken at "la pause" (tea break) one afternoon. I have it before me as I write. There we all are. Fat Vincent, who dunned me daily for fags. Roland, with his patch over one eye. Félicien making a silly "V" with his fingers behind Guillaume.

Pierre, Jean-Xavier, Philippe, Christine, Jean-Benoit looking (appropriately) like some South American bandito. Me, with my sandal visible on my chest. I took it warmly and thanked them all, trying to express in my broken French how much they had all meant to me. But they interrupted – I was to look on the back they said. So, I did, and tears jumped up to prick the back of my eyes.

They had all signed it. Some were well-scripted, nice messages of well-wishing, from Pierre for instance, and François. Most were not.

Most were shaky, schoolchild-like, scrawled signatures, nothing else. Philippe's, Vincent's, Jean-Xavier's, Guillaume's, Jean-Benoit's, one I can't even read.

I had never thought throughout the month that these fine people could not read or write. I had never distinguished between the literate and the illiterate. It had not mattered. And I realised, as my guts melted and I struggled to stop my face twisting into tears, that my lifetime's preoccupation with learning and the intellectual snobbery that goes with it had been a terrible prison. These grinning clowns looking at me now had shown me that. I was deep in their debt. If my house caught fire and I had time to save only one possession, it would be that photo. If I were to be asked what one piece of writing in all my reading had taught me the most it would be Roland's large, shaky, Elizabeth I-style signature in black biro on the back of that photo. Truly, the greatest work of L'Arche is for "those with learning difficulties". The surprise is that, more often than not, those who go to help are the ones who need to learn the most.

Thought for the Day

Moments of truth. Have you ever had a moment such as mine when I was given that photo? When the defences of a lifetime are pierced and the posturing you go in for is exposed. It smarts, yet you know it is deeply good. It releases and relaxes yet it is almost painful to move, so long have you been stuck there. It is frightening; you are terrified of losing the moment. It seems so ephemeral against the concrete of your ingrained habits, a butterfly soon flitting away or crushed. Take heart. God is at work in you. He will not suffer that work to fail. Why these epiphanies come so fleetingly I cannot guess, unless it's our stubborn exclusion of them. Go back to your moment. Try to recapture its importance. Pray again to the Father, even if now the emotions of your moment have gone, that his work of grace continues in you.

Prayer

Lord, how terrible is the way we humans wall ourselves up for year after year, away from you and your grace. I am sorry it takes a lot to break through to me. I guess it took the blood of Jesus to get through to us all. Have mercy Lord. Have mercy Lord. Forgive us Lord. Grant newness of life. Amen.

Bible Passages
Ephesians 2:14-17
Jesus breaking down barriers.

Romans 7:19-23
Being set free from slavery to old sinful habits of mind, to holiness.

For Meditation
"If I just touch his clothes, I will be healed." (Mark 5:28)

DAY TWENTY-SIX
Country Dancing

"Praise his name with dancing"

The last night of my stay coincided with the closure of La Rebellerie for the summer holidays. This was marked by a special final evening including a whole community meeting, an end-of-term Mass and, you've guessed it, a big barbecue. The meeting was the only time I saw all the community under one roof. I was surprised at the number of people there, especially the young families. I had been mainly among the working teams, whose members were mostly single. The families were large, often with four or five children. I thought of the financial sacrifice it must be to live on a community allowance or something (I never knew how it was all done, but I doubt if they got rich) with a large family. Then I thought how nice a place to grow up rural France must be, even if you took no part in the community's life; the open fields, the quiet villages.

There were farewells and presentations. Two or three foyer leaders were leaving. Gerhard was given his wine. I was surprised how muted the thanks were. Among these voluble French I would have thought more would have been said. At our local twinning affairs you can't shut the French town clerk up. But here it was just a quick word and then on with the next. And this after people had put in at least a year of unremitting hard work. There was very little fuss made at La Rebellerie.

The Mass was lovely, with everyone squeezed into the homely chapel. I was more prepared for not being able to receive the elements than last time, though it still bit.

Over the barbecue food I got to talk with M. Le Brun, the Director of La Rebellerie. He had only arrived at the community a few weeks previously. I was very impressed. I had expected a low-key conversation about travel and arrangements and so on. But he spoke of his faith, of what Jean Vanier had said to him, of his conversion from a nominal belief to a vibrant one. I asked what he had been doing before. I forget what it was now but he was a professionally qualified person and had left it to bring his young family to L'Arche. His eyes were firm and full of faith. I wished him well.

Then there was some country dancing, initiated by my old friend Roland, the local doctor, on a rickety cassette player. I am used to country dancing. It is a much-used thing in local church life. It is a great leveller – children and adult, agile and flatfooted, shy and extrovert – all can get along fine with it. That is why it is so much used in churches where you have to mix all manner of people. And it has charm.

This dancing was different. For a start, not everyone was dragooned into it. There was no repeated calling out for another couple to complete the set while we all stood around getting bored. Nor were there the endless rehearsals and walking through of the thing with everyone chiming out the steps like schoolchildren. Those who wished just got on and danced the dance, no messing. And such dances! Splendid, complex ones with the man and the woman, hip to hip, holding each other across their backs and cavorting like horses at play. Espérence and Guillaume, proud ones the both, formed a fine pair, Guillaume with his spare arm cocked to his outside hip like a flamenco dancer and Espérence tossing her chestnut hair. Philippe seized the fair

Agathe as a bear might seize a baby, wrapping his massive arm around the small of her back and whisking her away from the side of her astonished friend. She wore a smile throughout that showed she didn't mind. Pierre, competent at this as at all things, took his wife Sophie effortlessly through the interesting, heel and toe, half-kicking steps. All was not beauty however, some was comedy. Guy, who could scarcely walk without tripping over his big feet, lolloped about with the dainty Sally, who managed to dodge his worst clompings while performing creditably herself. And I thundered around with Nicole, Roland's wife.

At the end we stood there breathless, chests heaving, laughing. The evening sun shone slanting down, throwing our faces half into golden light, half into shadow. I looked around me. The cream buildings with their terracotta roofs, the grass and the pretty pond, the knots of people chatting, the broad sky approaching the gloaming, us dancers wondering whether to have one last dance. Suddenly a pang of pain lanced my side. I thought, "Tomorrow, I am leaving these people for good, and I don't want to. For all the drudgery, the flies, the unfamiliarity, my bad French, I don't want to go. Not even to my family, nor my beloved cranky parish. I don't want to leave."

And then there flooded in all the useless rationalisations. I would come back, I would keep in touch etc. Only, I wouldn't. This was the end. There was something desperately beautiful here. Clear and vital as water, and I was going back to thirsty normality. I wanted to throw over my normal life and join this community full time and maybe I should, maybe that was one of those defining moments when you should leap into the dark and not hesitate. But anyway, they were shutting for the holidays.

Thought for the Day

Think about the last time you danced. Where was it? And when? What were your feelings as you danced? How free did you feel to dance as you wished? Were you self-conscious? Who else was there? Perhaps it is many years since you danced? Perhaps you avoid it? Perhaps you would like to dance deep inside but feel too – too what? Too old? Too fat? Too silly? Too out of touch? Take some time before your God today to decide if it would please him if you danced in some context or another. Completely privately in worship maybe, or some other way. At one of our church socials recently, a man who had refused to dance with his wife throughout their thirty years of marriage, got up and offered to dance with her. It redefined their love. Maybe you need to take some similar step, redefining your love for your own body, perhaps, if for no one else.

Prayer

Lord my pride and my fear are terrible twins. They keep me living in a sterile state called normality which really suppresses most of who I am. No. It's not them. It's me. I am proud, hating to look silly. I am afraid, desperately afraid, all the time, of what others might think. I now choose to please you and to be myself. I will allow my soul, and my body to dance. Amen.

Bible Passage
2 Samuel 6:16-23
David dances before the Lord with all his might. Notice too the barrenness visited on Michal, who refuses to accept the dancing.

For Meditation
"Praise his name with dancing." (Psalm 149:3)

DAY TWENTY-SEVEN
Les Larmes de Compassion
(The Tears of Compassion)

"Jesus wept"

I t was my final morning at L'Arche and we were all in the morning
meeting. It was no less lively than usual. I had expected the half-
hour morning devotional meeting to be a decorous, quiet affair.
Certainly the brief reading and prayer, followed by the Lord's Prayer
all said together, were so. After that, though, came the announcements
for the day. Most of the time I could not follow these, so quick was the
French, but I followed the hooting and laughter that accompanied
them. The announcer was cheered on, his every word. Any slight slip
of the tongue caused gales of laughter, not derision, just amusement.
Every instruction affirmed with, "Oui chef. D'accord chef. Vraiment
chef" (Yes boss. OK boss. Sure boss) all around. There were comments
and ribaldry flying about all over the room. It was all very lively,
though completely mystifying to me.

This final day was going to see all at work until 4 p.m., even though
everybody was going to be gone on holiday by the evening. As
Thomas announced this I thought again how hard working and unfussy

these folks were. I felt strange sat there in ordinary day clothes, not my boiler suit, as I was needing to leave that morning, a long journey ahead of me. The meeting was soon over and everyone poured out of the room to their work. I had no need, as I was not going to work, so I stayed on in the room looking at the pleasing centrepiece for worship made by the scouts, taking some time to thank God for my experiences of the month. I suddenly realised I was not alone. Across the room was Jean-Benoit. I went to sit by him, to say goodbye, I imagine. He seemed unaware of me. He was away in a world of his own, as sometimes he would, just sitting there, his black olive eyes unfocussed. From some sudden impulse I lifted a hand and stroked his cheek. I can still remember the feel of the bristles under my fingertips. Then I went back to my place. And then the tears came. They spilled out of my eyes noiselessly like taps overflowing at first, running down my face as I sat still. Then big sobs followed, shaking my body. My old sparring partner Jean-Benoit sat on in his world. The scouts' centrepiece with its twisted wood and its cross hung wordlessly before me. And I cried, I knew not why. The door opened. I looked up blearily. It was Anne-Marie – who else? She gave a little grunt at seeing me so, much as when she had caught me in the shower.

"Ça va?" (You OK?)

I shrugged. She gave another grunt, standing there half round the door.

"Ce sont les larmes de compassion" (They are the tears of compassion.)

And then she was gone. Again no fuss. At my church somebody in my state would have had a knot of people hovering around like fire-tenders mopping them up. Here – this quick, kind comment, a wry smile, and on with the job. Tears of compassion. Were they? I hope so. I know I was glad to shed them.

The last I saw of Jean-Benoit was him sitting there still. Though there was a post-script. On my return from my own holiday a month later, was a letter. It was from him. It said simply,

"André, tu me manques", (Andrew, I miss you.)

I think he wrote so to all the assistants and I doubt if he misses me now. But I miss him, that's for sure.

Thought for the Day

Tears of compassion. Tears can be many things can they not? They can be self-pity, moral blackmail, delaying tactics, attention-seeking, nostalgia, maudlin sentimentality, to name but a few. And I guess they can be pure from time to time. Perhaps when we are surprised by our tears is when they are at their best. Think over your own tears. Or your lack of them. Sometimes we are beyond them. I recall the funeral I took of a young man of twenty-one – the only son of his single mother. Hers were the only dry eyes in the church. She was beyond tears. Ask God for tears of compassion.

Prayer

Lord, let me cry
And when I do,
Let my tears
Be of You.
Amen.

Bible Passage
Ezra 3:10-13
The weeping mixed with joy at the refounding of the temple.

For Meditation
"Jesus wept." (John 11:35)

DAY TWENTY-EIGHT

La Porte est Grande Ouverte
(The Door is Wide Open)

"Open wide your mouth and I will fill it"

Once I had left Jean-Benoit to his thoughts I made my way to the office to pay my phone bill and buy some cases of La Rebellerie's own produce to take home. Then I returned to the foyer to pack and stow my bags into my little grey car. The cases of wine were too heavy to carry back to the foyer so I had arranged to drive down to the centre to collect them before leaving for home.

This caused me to take a different exit road from the complex than I otherwise would and it furnished the happy chance that I would unexpectedly pass the vines team at work weeding around some newly planted vines. I saw them before they saw me: their work looked backbreaking as usual and I have to say I didn't mind leaving that behind one little bit. Then one of them looked up, Philippe I think, and saw my car. He immediately gave out a red indian-style whoop and came galumphing down the field towards me. The others, too, looked up and, once they realised what was afoot, came on apace, until they were circling my car in true Western fashion. I had stopped and wound down my window for one last farewell. In no time my windscreen wipers were going and the screen was covered in foamy water, my hazard lights were winking, my horn was being sounded, hands were reaching in to flick open the glove compartment, my tube of sweets for the journey was being handed round. It was happy mayhem. I sat blinking around in the midst of this, trying to get my bearings, when suddenly my two ears were grasped at their roots by strong hands and my head was twisted round to face out of the car. Félicien held me there a moment for a considered look at me, then he put his face right into mine, his eyes one inch away. I wondered what he would say. He said, in a voice of surprising tenderness, given the rough treatment of just now, "Reviens, André, la porte est grande ouverte." (Come back sometime, Andrew, the door is wide open.)

It was the same as he had written on the back of my farewell photo. Perhaps he said it as a matter of course to all the assistants. It was important to remember that, while we came and went through La Rebellerie, for Félicien and the others it was permanent home. But still it stayed with me, his phrase, during all the long miles to my home. The door is wide open. It would make not a bad motto for L'Arche. Jean Vanier opened his doors once and his movement still keeps them open. Open to people like Félicien, who could thank them for a new life. Open to people like me, who could thank them for a new outlook. Open to God, who will thank them for valuing that which the world rejects and making it the cornerstone of a truly beautiful temple to his name.

Thought for the Day

Try applying "The door is wide open" to your life. How well does it fit? Think of times when you have opened a door in your life to someone else – particularly where that was risky. What was the outcome? Did it prove a doorway to something important and good?

Did you regret it? Are there areas of life where you are shutting your doors? Are you keeping out of your life any people who God wants in it? Are you on the whole a guarded person or an open one? Big questions, but it was through answering them that L'Arche came into being.

Prayer

Lord, help me never to forget that I can come to you only because you kindly grant access to the undeserving. You open your doors wide indeed. Forgive me my tight, shut-up-shop, keep-what's-mine attitude. Open me up please. I am aware you will need to prise me like a clam, but I will try to be cooperative. And I know that only by going through this can I truly be free. Amen.

Bible Passages
Numbers 14
This passage is about the dangers of refusing to enter open doors. The people of Israel refuse to enter the Promised Land. For a commentary on this read Hebrews 4:1-13.

For Meditation
"Here I am! I stand at the door and knock. If anyone hears my voice and opens the door, I will come in and eat with him, and he with me." (Revelation 3:20)

"Open wide your mouth and I will fill it." (Psalm 81:10)

Epilogue

I hope you enjoyed using these devotions. If you wish to know anything further about L'Arche, their UK details are:

L'Arche Secretariat
10 Briggate
Silsden
Keighley
West Yorkshire
BD20 9JT

Telephone: +44 (0)1535 656186
Fax: +44 (0)1535 656426
E-mail: info@larche.org.uk
Website address: www.larche.org.uk

The community at La Rebellerie are also happy to be contacted. Their details are:

La Rebellerie
49560
Nueil-sur-Layon
FRANCE

Telephone: +33 (0)2 41 59 53 51
+33 (0)2 41 59 99 89
E-mail: larebellerie.rc@larchefrance.org
Website address: perso.wanadoo.fr/arche.rebellerie
www.larchefrance.org

You may like to try for yourself the method I used to write each day's piece. It is not difficult and, for me, has proved a great way into appreciating how God is at work in my very ordinary, everyday life. I so often pine for him to reveal himself more to me when all along, there in my day-to-day existence, are all kinds of epiphanies small and great – if I would just slow down and take the time to appreciate them.

Here is the recipe if you want it.

1. Look back at your day or some comparable period. Decide what struck you the most about it.

2. Write about that facet of your experience in full. Don't try to be all literary. Just write as if you were sharing it over coffee with a close friend. You will nearly always be surprised, once you start, just how rich and evocative your experience was. Also, how deep and subtle were your reactions.

3. Later, probably the next day, reflect on your experience and think over in what ways the incident you describe connects with your Christian faith. Write a piece about that too. Not too long. Just a basic thought or two.

4. Try to find a portion of scripture which connects your experience. If you are stuck, use a concordance or similar Bible guide. Ponder over the links between the scripture passage and your piece of living. Write a thought or two on it.

5. Write a prayer. Use you own words. Say to God exactly what you feel. Don't censor it. Don't worry about offending him – he's got a thick skin. He loves you and is glad of any sincere prayer. And he will answer with great power.

6. Pick a key phrase from out of it all, probably from the Bible and take ten minutes to meditate on it, swirling it around your spirit like a wine taster swirling wine around a glass.

You may be intrigued to know that what you have just done is some "practical theology", an increasingly recognised way of discovering God. They even have university professorships in it. You start from everyday life, think into it and then forge some connections between it and the historic faith. This is in distinction from the more conventional method of starting with scripture and tradition and applying it to our everyday life. I reckon we all hurtle through life, gobbling down its nourishment without remotely taking the time and thoughtfulness to appreciate just how much God is giving of himself to us every single day of our lives. It is good to take stock in this way, to use the written word – so sacred a thing – and dwell on the wonderful love of God shown to us in new ways every day. And, sometimes, we can be yearning for God to reveal himself to us and be, perhaps, working too hard at our conventional devotions, when, if we stop and ponder like this just on our ordinary existence – there is God, waiting to be met.